Psychology Revivals

The A B C of Nerves

Originally published in 1928, the preface reads: "It is almost impossible to distinguish between what is 'elementary' and what is 'advanced' in regard to the nervous system. The constitution and functions of that system are so little matters of common knowledge that it would be safe to assume that practically nothing of its physiology is known to the ordinary reader.

The selection of what is necessary to be known and likely to be comprehended by readers who have no previous knowledge of anatomy and physiology is, therefore, no easy task.

It is certain that in the opinion of some authorities much has been omitted that should have been included; one can but say in self-defence that to have included more than is here considered would have exceeded the limits of a treatise whose title is the A B C." Today it can be read and enjoyed in its historical context.

The A B C of Nerves

D.F. Fraser-Harris

Routledge
Taylor & Francis Group
LONDON AND NEW YORK

First published in 1928
by Kegan Paul, Trench, Trubner & Co. Ltd

This edition first published in 2015 by Psychology Press

Published 2023 by Routledge
4 Park Square, Milton Park, Abingdon, Oxon OX14 4RN
605 Third Avenue, New York, NY 10017

Routledge is an imprint of the Taylor & Francis Group, an informa business

Publisher's Note
The publisher has gone to great lengths to ensure the quality of this reprint but points out that some imperfections in the original copies may be apparent.

Disclaimer
The publisher has made every effort to trace copyright holders and welcomes correspondence from those they have been unable to contact.

A Library of Congress record exists under LCCN: 29027519

ISBN: 978-1-138-93030-8 (hbk)
ISBN: 978-1-315-68025-5 (ebk)

THE ABC OF NERVES

BY

D. F. FRASER-HARRIS

M.D., D.Sc., F.R.S.E.

LONDON

KEGAN PAUL, TRENCH, TRUBNER & CO., LTD

BROADWAY HOUSE : 68-74 CARTER LANE, E.C.

1928

MADE AND PRINTED IN GREAT BRITAIN BY
M. F. ROBINSON & CO., LTD., AT THE LIBRARY PRESS LOWESTOFT

TO

ALEC

ONE OF THE MERRIEST

CONTENTS

FIGURES IN THE TEXT

[illegible]

[illegible]

[illegible]

[illegible]

[illegible]

[illegible]

[illegible]

[illegible]

[illegible]

[illegible]

[illegible]

[illegible]

[illegible]

[illegible]

[illegible]

PREFACE

It is almost impossible to distinguish between what is " elementary " and what is " advanced " in regard to the nervous system. The constitution and functions of that system are so little matters of common knowledge that it would be safe to assume that practically nothing of its physiology is known to the ordinary reader.

The selection of what is necessary to be known and likely to be comprehended by readers who have no previous knowledge of anatomy and physiology is, therefore, no easy task.

It is certain that in the opinion of some authorities much has been omitted that should have been included ; one can but say in self-defence that to have included more than is here considered would have exceeded the limits of a treatise whose title is the A B C.

LONDON, D. F. F-H.

October, 1928.

A B C OF NERVES

CHAPTER I

THE PRE-EMINENCE OF THE NERVOUS SYSTEM

It is usual to speak of the nervous system as the noblest of the systems in the body. The chief systems composing the body are: the skeletal, the muscular, the circulatory, the digestive, the respiratory, the excretory, and the nervous.

The bodily frame consists of bones and joints, muscles to move these, digestive organs to prepare food for absorption, blood in blood-vessels to carry that nourishment to all parts, the respiratory system to introduce oxygen, a gaseous food, and to eliminate carbon-dioxide and water, the excretory glands to get rid of soluble waste matter, and lastly the nervous system to control all the others.

The nervous system, the most important in its activities, is perhaps the least obvious

C

and most inaccessible of the great systems. Everybody knows what a bone is like; we all know what muscle or flesh is like; but few people are so familiar with the brain, the spinal cord or the nerves. There is a dish, "sheep's head with brain-cakes", more often seen in Scotland than in England, but not now to be had much even there, in which we may see a brain cooked; but we rarely see a nerve, and when we do, we may easily mistake it for a tendon (sinew), as did the ancient Greeks, whose word *neuron* meant a tendon, but now means a nerve. The central nervous system is the most perfectly protected system in the body. The brain (cerebrum) and cerebellum are protected by the hard bones of the skull; and the spinal cord is in the interior of what is called the back-bone, which is really a column of small bones possessing a central canal in which the cord is lodged.

The word "brain", being a popular term, is a vague one. Anatomists use the term Encephalon for the whole contents of the skull, and the encephalon includes the cerebrum (or brain), the cerebellum, and the "Bulb", the lower part of which is called the Medulla Oblongata.

The medulla oblongata can be looked upon as the upward extension of the spinal cord, for there is no real line of separation between the two.[1]

The Bulb contains a number of what are called vital "centres", groups of nerve-cells presiding over certain important bodily activities. Some of these centres are: the centre which regulates breathing; that which regulates the action of the heart; the centre for regulating the calibre of the blood-vessels; the centres for the glands of the alimentary canal; the vomiting centre; the centre for perspiration, and others. We shall later learn exactly what a "centre" is. Centres are the essence of the nervous system; they correspond to railway stations, the nerves to railway lines; the one without the other is of no use. Just as certain lines come into a railway station and others leave it, so certain nerves lead into centres and other lead out of them. Nerves connected with no centres would be as useless as railway lines connected with no stations. Stations also are clearly of no use by themselves.

Why is the nervous system called the most

[1] The central nervous system is that part contained within the skull and vertebral column, the peripheral nervous system is all the rest.

noble or master system? Because it is the more or less active overseer of all parts of the body: it controls or influences the muscles, the heart, the blood-vessels, the glands, and the movements of breathing, of the alimentary canal, and of other internal organs. To do this effectively the nervous system must be receiving information from as many parts as possible. The nerves of the peripheral nervous system are the totality of the ingoing and outgoing channels of communication; the centres are the places to which and from which the nerves proceed.

This being-attended-to-by-the-nervous-system is called in physiology *innervation*, or the condition of being innervated.[1] A good example of the working of the nervous system is that of the telephone exchange of a great city. The girls and their switch-boards are the centres, the ingoing wires are the sensory nerves, the outgoing wires are the motor nerves. The central exchange connects the two people A and B who want to talk to each other. They may live next door, that is of no consequence; if they

[1] The word "innervated" should be distinguished from "enervated", which means tired out.

want to talk to each other, they must still do so through the "central" which may be a mile away. Thus, when the mischievous school-boy sticks a pin into the toe of his unsuspecting friend, and the foot of the latter gives a sudden violent jerk, the stabbed nerves of the skin of the toe sent a message all the way up to nerve-cells in the spinal cord whence fresh messages were sent down all the way to the muscles of the foot to cause them to contract. This is the kind of thing we shall later learn to call a "reflex action".

Other examples are: the mouth "watering" when an acid such as vinegar is applied to the tongue, sneezing when something tickles the nose, coughing when something tickles the windpipe, having a hiccough when something irritates the stomach, and so forth.

Clearly a centre must both receive and transmit; the girl receives a message from A, and she adjusts matters in the "centre" so that A is put in communication with B; "the central" or centre is indispensable. One might say that the girl's ears were a receiving centre and her hands an emitting centre, that is to say, she is two related centres. Such an arrangement undoubtedly occurs in the nervous system; one centre is receptive, while a closely related one is emissive.

Take the case of speech; we hear words, we reply by words; we receive, we give out. The complete neural mechanism of speech involves sensory or receptive centres and motor or emissive ones. We hear words, we have ideas, and we express them in words. Some of the speech-centres are the physical basis of the comprehension of heard or of seen words, these are the sensory speech-centres; while others are *for* actuating the muscles of articulation, and others *for* the hand in writing. Were it not for these "centres" there would be nothing to connect the sounds we call words with the appropriate muscular movements we call speech; and if there were no centres, the heard or seen words would call up no meanings, would never give rise to any ideas. But the nervous system resembles closely a vast organization like an army in the field. Just as in the army there are degrees of responsibility, each person lower down being responsible to some one higher up until we come to the commander-in-chief. Any one holding a rank gives orders to those below him and takes orders from those above him. It is the same in the nervous system; centres receive from those above them and discharge to those below them. There is, as it is called, a hierarchy of centres, for centres are by no means all on the same functional level.

The private soldiers correspond to the muscles which do all the actual, ultimate moving of things, for, as has been truly said, in the last analysis we can only move things; the officers are the nerve-centres originating the commands which the soldiers execute; the nerve-fibres are the means of communication between officers and men.

Thus we speak of the nervous system as the system which controls; it controls and influences all the others. Under this aspect the nervous system is the "highest" or most noble, the others are "lower"; and within the nervous system there are degrees of power or eminence, just as there are in the Church and in the Army where the bishop is above the curate and the general above the lieutenant.

It should be noted very clearly that the centres of the nervous system receive no energy from the impulses reaching them from the sense organs. Just as the officers' orders give the rank and file no energy wherewith to carry them out, so the stimulations arriving in the nervous system confer no energy upon the centres for their output of impulses. The soldiers get their energy for their marching from the food they consume, so the nervous system gets its energy—like every other system—from the food it assimilates. This is, of course, the physiology of the military dictum that "an army marches on its stomach", no transcendental discovery, for all work is done on food consumed.

Potential energy is stored by the centres of the nervous system, and the stimuli from outside impinging on these centres merely release the energy in the active or kinetic form. Neural stimuli are the means of making patent the energy that is already latent in the nervous system; they are not energy-producing in themselves. Such stimuli are often called "releasing" stimuli.

The words of command are the appropriate stimuli for the soldiers to exhibit the energy that may be in them; but the commands confer no energy; that is the concern of the Commissariat. And just as the soldiers *could* act of themselves were there no officers present, so the centres can discharge impulses spontaneously. We shall see later that these spontaneous activities require guiding and controlling. All stimuli do not necessarily incite to action; some restrain or inhibit, as it is called; but in neither case do the stimuli give any power; they only liberate or restrain it. The mistake of imagining that stimulation gives power is a very widespread popular misconception.

There is a further analogy between the nervous system and the Army. The soldiers must be drilled, exercised, and disciplined, else in a short time they become "slack" and untidy; they may perform their duties, but in their own way and in their own time. The cessation of commands leads to lack of discipline and to disorganization. Innervation means that each man knows he is being thought of at headquarters, and so virtually he is, for so long as "the orders for the day" come through, each man feels he is not forgotten.

In order that a regiment may be ready for any emergency on the shortest notice, it must be drilled frequently and each man must know his place and his duty. Now to all this there is a close analogy in the nervous system; the nerve-impulses continually descending upon the muscles keep them in good condition, firm, " tonic " as it is called, for very shortly after the nerves are cut, the muscles, unable to be used, suffer from disuse, from atrophy, and become flabby and watery. They are no longer innervated, drilled, held in readiness, toned up by the nervous impulses; they are on the contrary *a*tonic.

Muscles properly innervated are ready to respond to the stimulus to go into activity with the minimum of delay, the exceedingly short period of delay between the moment of the reception of the impulse and the beginning of the contraction is called the " latent period ".

Further, the various units, e.g. regiments, of an army have quite definite places and duties in the field; they have relationships to one another just as the individual members of the rank and file have. This is absolutely necessary for effective co-operation in battle: some one must know what the various units have to do and where exactly they are doing it. In action, the orders which originate from headquarters are ultimately transmitted to each man, and the battle develops according to the scheme of the commander-in-chief. But if the communications are interfered with and the men cut off from their officers, the fight develops into what is called a "soldier's battle". The men are individually as strong and as intelligent as before, but each man fights by himself and not with regard to orders from above nor with regard to what his neighbour is doing; the co-ordination of man with man and regiment with regiment is lost, and the battle will almost always be more or less of a chaos. A victory may be won, but it will be rather by luck than by skill. Co-ordinated action is the keynote of a successful engagement.

The analogy of all this with the working of the nervous system is very close. When muscles are no longer in their normal relationships to their centres, then they cease to be in good tone; they are not properly related to one another, in fact are not co-ordinated.

There is still another aspect which shows the functional superiority of the nervous system. If an animal be deprived of food but given water, it can, as is well known, survive for some weeks, but dies when its total loss of weight amounts to about a half or two-thirds of the initial.

Two cats of the same age and weight were taken; one was deprived of all food, and the other killed in order to estimate the weights of the different organs before starvation was endured.[1] When the starving cat died, its organs were weighed, and it was found that whereas the fat had completely disappeared and the muscles had wasted to 42.2% of their original weight, the heart and the nervous system had practically not wasted at all. The skin had lost 8.8, the bones 5.4, the liver 4.8, and the blood 3.7% respectively of their original weights. This shows how functionally important are the heart and the nervous system; without the integrity of both of them, life could not be maintained. The fat and the muscles have actually been digested (by a process known as autolysis), and the products of that digestion have been carried in the blood to feed the heart and nervous system. Thus there is feeding in starvation, so that Shakespeare is right when he says,

> "I sup upon myself and so shall starve with feeding"
> (*Coriolanus*, iv. 2).

Clearly the nervous system is the ruling

[1] These experiments were made eighty years ago by the Frenchman Chossat, and fortunately do not need to be repeated.

system, and if so it must be fed at all costs. All other systems are subservient to it. Even when there is no food for the lower systems, they must provide food for the higher; and such is the inexorable necessity of the higher, that the lower actually give themselves up to feed this master-tissue.

Lastly, as indicating the eminence in the hierarchy of systems to which the nervous has attained, we may point to the arrangements for the maintenance of its blood-supply. As is well known to anatomists, the arteries at the base of the brain which are supplied chiefly from the two great carotids, form a large hexagonal meeting-place, the "Circle of Willis". This is so constructed that if one limb of the hexagon is blocked up, for instance by a blood-clot, the supply of blood to the brain would still be adequate, through the other five limbs. But further than this, the blood supply is so arranged that if more blood is required in the cerebral vessels, it is obtained by the vessels of the abdomen being constricted and thus forcing to the head the blood so shut out from the internal organs. This reciprocal arrangement is governed from a centre in the medulla oblongata itself. The medulla oblongata has a supply from a separate source, the basilar artery; so that blocking up of the carotids would still leave a supply of blood to the extremely important Bulb.

The original illustration of this "circle" (really hexagon) of Willis, along with many other figures, was drawn by Christopher Wren for Willis's book on the anatomy of the brain published in 1680.

The capillaries of the nervous system are conveyed to it in delicate connective tissue called the pia mater which closely ensheathes the entire nervous system. Over the cortex it dips down into the folds or sulci which are found between the convolutions or gyri. It is excessively vascular. Curiously enough this membrane is mentioned three times in the plays of Shakespeare.

The first is in a speech by Holofernes in *Love's Labour Lost*, where he says of ideas that "these are begot in the ventricle of memory, nourished in the womb of pia mater, and delivered upon the mellowing of occasion" (IV. 2).

We cannot suppose that Shakespeare knew anatomy to the extent of understanding that the pia mater, by conveying to the brain its nutrient blood-vessels, does literally nourish the brain, and therefore may be said to nourish things like ideas which are the results of the activity of the brain.

The pia mater is mentioned twice more; in *Twelfth Night* (I. 5) and in *Troilus and Cressida* (II. 1). It has been suggested that Shakespeare got his anatomical terms out of a text-book of Anatomy he might have picked up at Jaggard's book-shop in the Barbican, seeing that Jaggard was his own printer. In this book (Anatomy by Helkiah Crooke), the pia mater has a very prominent place.

CHAPTER II

THE CONSTITUTION AND ARCHITECTURE OF THE NERVOUS SYSTEM

(1) NERVE-CELLS AND NERVE-FIBRES

Every nerve-fibre is the living out-growth or "process" of a living nerve-cell, and functionally one is of no use without the other. Each nerve-cell gives rise to one nerve-fibre intended for some definite destination.

Individual nerve-cells and nerve-fibres are invisible because they are microscopically small.[1] But thousands of nerve-fibres bound together into the "nerve-trunk", as anatomists call it, are visible in the mass, and being covered with a glistening connective tissue sheath *do* resemble a tendon. A tendon is, however, much denser and tougher than a nerve-trunk. The old name for nerve-

[1] There is one exception to this, the nerve-cell of the electric organ of one of the electric fishes which is just visible to the unaided eye.

cells was grey matter, for nerve-fibres, white matter.

If, by appropriate means, we disintegrate a nerve-trunk, we can make out under the microscope that it consists of a very large number of exceedingly minute, opaque, soft, pale grey cylinders or fibres held together by a quantity of delicate tissue known to anatomists as "connective". Thus the individual fibres are separated from one another like a number of tall bottles would be if packed upright in a box and prevented from touching one another by the "packing" of cotton wool or straw.

If we cut an inch or so off one of these nerves and "fix" it by placing it in some chemical solution which prevents changes in its structure and composition, "harden" it by appropriate means, cut it into extremely thin "sections" across the fibres, and then look at these (duly stained) under the microscope, we shall be able to notice the following details—(1) a tiny central core, evidently the transverse section of a central thread which is called the axis-cylinder or neuraxon; (2) an opaque white fatty sheath called the medullary sheath; and (3) an outermost, excessively thin sheath, the neurilemma. Because of the presence of the fatty sheath, a fibre of this kind is called a medullated nerve-fibre.

The transverse section of a nerve-trunk is so like that of an electric cable that the resemblance has frequently been remarked on: the conducting strand, the axis-cylinder corresponds to the copper wire itself, while the medullary sheath answers to the gutta-percha or other insulating material. Just as the electric current travels in the copper wire and not in the insulation, so the nerve-impulses travel in the axis-cylinder and not in the connective tissue.[1]

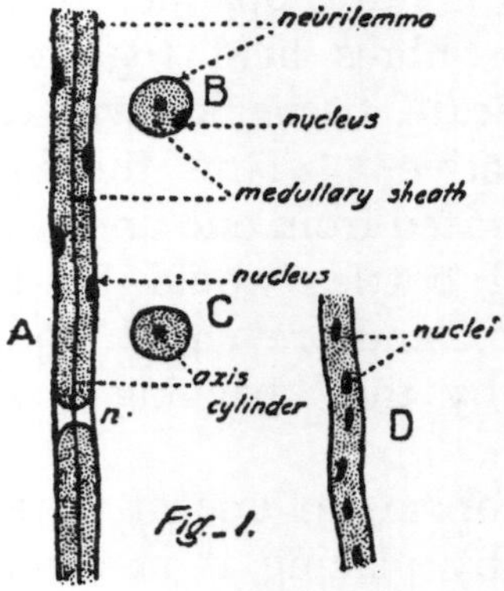

Nerve Fibres (highly magnified).

A. Medullated fibre, longitudinal view.
B. Medullated fibre, transverse view.
C. White fibre from central nervous system, transverse section.
D. Non-medullated fibre, longitudinal view.
n. Node, or place where medullary sheath is interrupted.

[1] Not all nerve-fibres possess a fatty sheath: there are some nerves which have only an axis-cylinder and nuclei and are therefore called *non*-medullated fibres. The nuclei appear as swellings on a clear, ribbon-like fibre, which from its appearance is called a pale fibre or fibre of Remak after its discoverer, a German physician, Robert Remak (1815-1865).

It is now certainly known that the central axis-cylinder is the outgrowth of some nerve-cell; it is the long delicate conducting fibre which owes its origin and life to the presence of the cell. The fatty sheath contributes in some way to the maintenance of

Fig. 2.

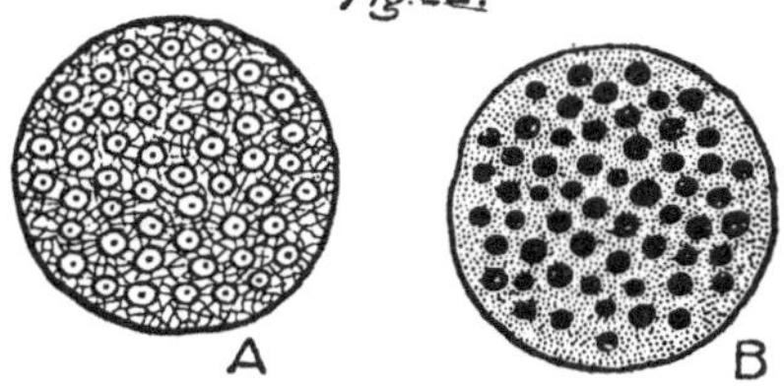

A. Transverse section of a nerve bundle, the individual medullated nerves are seen surrounded by "connective tissue".
B. Transverse section of an electric cable, the individual wires are seen surrounded by insulating material.

the life of the axis-cylinder, but the cell alone produced the latter and alone can reproduce it. It was found that if a nerve-fibre is severed from its cell of origin, the cell lives while the fibre dies. The piece of fibre still attached to the cell-body begins after an interval to grow towards the periphery.[1]

[1] The word "periphery" in this connexion means all parts of the body beyond (outside of) the central nervous system.

These facts discovered by A. V. Waller, 1850 (1816-1870) are known as Wallerian Degeneration and Wallerian Regeneration. Wallerian Degeneration has been found to be of the utmost value to neurologists trying to discover which groups of nerve-cells (ganglia or nuclei) were related to particular strands of white fibres often not at all near to the cells in question. The problem frequently is to determine where fibres, originating in certain cells, end. This method gives us a means of tracing fibres which have died after severance from their "trophic" cells, because as seen under the microscope they stain differently from living ones.

The phenomenon of Wallerian degeneration is not an isolated one. It is well known to biologists that if a single nucleated cell be cut into two portions, so that one retains the nucleus[1] and the other does not, only the former continues to live. While the non-nucleated portion of the cell dies, the nucleated portion not only lives but reconstitutes the injured cell.

That portion of the nerve fibre, severed from the cell, dies throughout its entire length. Under the microscope one can see that the

[1] The nucleus is the central essential portion of every cell.

homogenous axis-cylinder and fatty sheath have become broken up into fatty globules which in time are more or less perfectly removed by white blood corpuscles.

While a nerve-cell and its attached stump can make that stump grow out towards the periphery as a new medullated fibre, a nerve-cell destroyed is not made good by the compensatory cell-division and growth of neighbouring nerve-cells, as is the case, for instance, with the skin or with bone, in both of which the powers of repair are highly developed.

(2) SOME TYPES OF CELLS OF THE CENTRAL NERVOUS SYSTEM

No elements of the human body as seen by the microscope assume so many forms as do nerve-cells. In common with all cells, each has a mass of protoplasm (cell-body), surrounding a nucleus. Some cells have quite smooth bodies. In this case there is but one process at each " pole ", as it is called, so that the old name for this type of cell was " bi-polar ".

It is convenient to have one word to describe the cell-body and all its processes whatsoever ; the word " neuron " is now used.

The neuron C has, therefore, a peripheral process A beginning in an arborescence *a*, and a central process B ending in an arborescence *b*. In the human body this type of afferent neuron is found only in the nerve supplying the ear, the auditory nerve (the eighth cranial), but in many lower animal forms, it is the prevailing type of neuron.

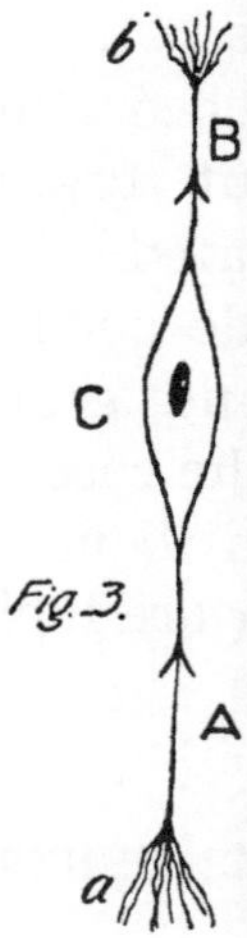

A " bi-polar neuron ".

C is the nucleated cell-body.
A and B are processes.
a and *b* arborescences.

The next type of cell is closely allied to the bi-polar, it is described as the cell with the T-shaped junction (Fig. 4). It differs from the previous type only in that the cell-body is placed on one side of the process. This always afferent neuron is found very widely distributed amongst the nerves, for it is the type present in every mixed[1] spinal nerve, and in the great sensory nerve of the face and head (Fifth cranial).

[1]A mixed nerve is one which contains both sensory and motor fibres.

The length of the neuron may be several feet, for it may arise in the skin of the sole of the foot and pass up one of the mixed nerves of the leg through the posterior root into the spinal cord where it may travel as far as the medulla oblongata in the neck. Thus some neurons, although of microscopic transverse dimensions, may yet be from four to five feet in length.

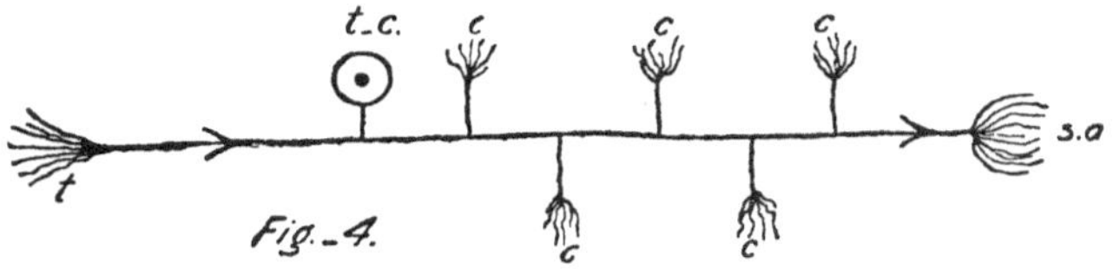

Diagram of a single afferent neuron (as in the Fifth Cranial nerve).

t.c. trophic cell with T-shaped junction.
t. arborescence of origin, say, in skin (peripheral).
c collaterals with arborizations for synapses.
s.a. terminal central synaptic arborization.

The third type of nerve-cell we must notice is an efferent or motor one; the type found in the anterior grey matter of the spinal cord. The cell-body has dendrites, and gives origin to a very long axis-cylinder process which, as soon as it has left the cord, becomes the axis-cylinder of a medullated motor nerve-fibre. Fig. 5 shows the neuron diagrammatically.

A fourth type of neuron is that found in

the grey matter of the brain (cortex cerebri).

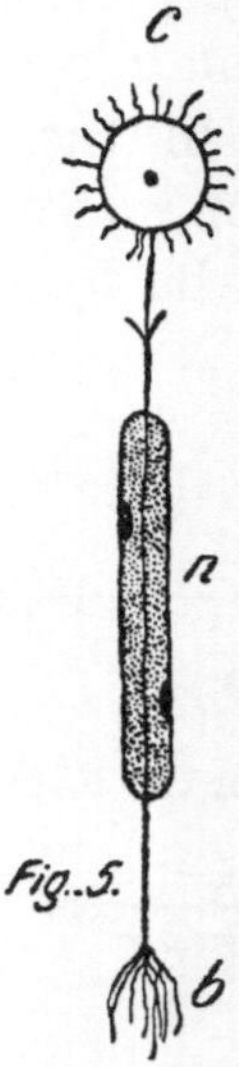

Diagram of motor neuron in spinal cord.

C, cell-body with dendrites (*d*) trophic for the nerve ; (*n*) is the motor-nerve which may be two or three feet long (the parts in the diagram are out of proportion).

b termination of nerve on muscle (not represented). This type used to be called "multipolar" on account of the dendrites (*d*).

The medullary sheath does not begin for some distance from the cell (C) and ends a short distance before the muscle is reached.

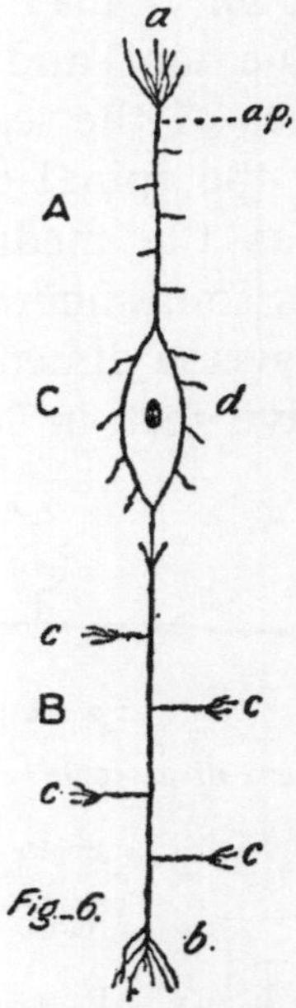

(Diagrammatic). Type of chief neuron from Cortex cerebri : (Golgi cell, type I).

C. nucleated trophic cell-body with dendrites *d*.

a is the apical arborescence *a.p.* apical process.

B neuraxon of medullated fibre (medullation not shown).

c collaterals ending in arborescences for synapses.

b terminal arborescence.

It is the most highly differentiated of all the nerve-cells. In addition to dendrites (*d*), it has an apical process (A) which begins in an arborescence (*a*); the neuraxon (B) which is medullated has medullated collaterals (*c*) each of which terminates in an arborescence (Fig. 6).

The neurons of this type we shall learn to call the upper motor neurons, and hence the cortex cerebri has been called the " highest trophic realm ". The shape of these cells is pyramidal; but curiously enough, that is not the reason why the tract of fibres emerging from these cells is called in the cord the (crossed) " pyramidal tract ". The reason is that the place of crossing of these upper neurons is called by anatomists the " decussation of the anterior pyramids ". The length of one of these pyramidal neurons may be very considerable, for it arises in the brain and may not terminate until quite low down in the region of the spinal cord where the motor-nerves for the muscles of the toes, for instance, originate. Thus, this neuron may be about three feet long.

The immature nerve-cell is known as a Neuroblast. It begins as a minute naked cell with the simplest possible apical process and neuraxon. Later, all the complexities of the fully developed neuron appear—dendrites, collaterals and arborescences at the synapses. (See page 30).

It is believed that collaterals can continue to be produced almost up to middle life (forty years), which means that fresh functional relationships on the part of the neuron can be entered into. One can easily see that this multiplication of collaterals and their connections with other neurons is the physiological basis of association of ideas and of educability. The demonstration of the existence of collaterals was a very important discovery. Fig. 4 shows us that by means of collaterals, nerve-impulses can be distributed to a great many structures other than those at the terminations of the main neuraxon. Through its collaterals (*c*), a single neuron can influence a very large number of other neurons which is the physical basis of such phenomena as co-ordination, spread of effects, and irradiation.

(3) EFFECTORS AND RECEPTORS

A convenient terminology in regard to peripheral tissues related to efferent and to afferent neurons was introduced by

Sir Charles Sherrington, F.R.S., some years ago.

Effectors. By an effector is meant any tissue which may receive nerve-impulses through an efferent nerve and thus give effect to them. The muscles are the most familiar receptors ; but the heart, the circular muscle of the small arteries and the various glands are other types of effector.

The muscle of the internal organs, the delicate muscles in the iris and other small muscles in the eye are all effectors. In the lower animals, the electric organ, the pigment cells of the skin, and the light-producing apparatus are also effectors.

Receptors. By a receptor is meant a particular kind of cell specialized to receive and be affected by some one kind of stimulus. These stimuli are the various forms of energy operating in the outer world—light, sound, heat and pressure as well as substances capable of being tasted or smelt. Receptors of this group are called extero-ceptors. All receptors are connected with the origins of afferent nerves.

The presence of the appropriate receptor as an intermediary between the stimulus and the nerve-fibre is imperative if the appropriate form of sensation is to develop. Thus, if the rods and cones, the receptors for light in the retina, are absent at any spot no light is perceived there. There is a form of blindness in which since these receptors are destroyed in patches in the retina, the patches are blind. Similarly when the end-organs have been overstimulated and are paralyzed, there is no normal sensation. This occurs in the eye in snow-blindness when the receptors in the retina are so damaged by the bright light that they cannot for a time perform their functions.

The functions of these receptors—formerly called "end-organs"—is to transmute the stimulus into that which will affect the sensory nerve-fibres.

If the cells of the epidermis of the skin are removed or destroyed, contact of the exposed nerve-fibrils gives rise not to a sensation of touch but to one of pain. Even a breath is painful to a blister, which is a place where there are no receptors for touch and where the nerves are exposed. Precisely the same is true of the teeth. When the enamel is intact we get certain sensations of resistance offered to our chewing efforts, when the enamel is undermined and the nerve below it in the interior of the tooth exposed, then we experience only pain.

A special term is used for the receptors found in the tissues themselves. For instance, embedded in muscle there are receptors stimulated by pressures, strains, torsions, etc., occurring in the muscles. Sherrington calls these "proprio-ceptors". The end-organs in the semi-circular canals of the internal ear are also classified as "proprio-ceptors", seeing that the stimuli effective here are not any changes of environmental energy but varying states of pressure in the fluid in these canals. On this terminology, the inter-nuncial neurons are called "connectors".

(4) CHROMATOLYSIS

This term refers to certain appearances seen under the microscope which develop in nerve-cells when they become abnormal in regard to their nutrition or function. All healthy nerve-cells, as stained and prepared for the microscope, show certain minute, rod-like bodies called "Granules of Nissl" after a German neurologist of that name. These granules show signs of being dissolved in a number of instances, the best known of which is fatigue. Prolonged activity evidently leads to this material being used up, whereas rest permits it to be reconstituted. Since it stains deeply it is called " chromatic " material, and when it undergoes solution or destruction the process is called " chromatolysis ".

This chromatolysis occurs also in cases where the cell has been poisoned by various deleterious substances.

Further, in certain diseases of the brain underlying mania and in some other forms of mental disease, the granules of Nissl are found more or less destroyed.

Finally, when for any reason the cell is not able to emit impulses into its neuraxon, it may show signs of chromatolysis which is only a particular case of " disuse atrophy ".

(5) SYNAPSES

The place where one neuron ends and the next begins, is one of great physiological importance, it is called a synapsis. Owing to the extreme delicacy of the living material at the origin of afferent neurons, and at the terminations of efferent neurons, and at those places called synapses, these regions are first and most seriously affected by poisons of all sorts circulating in the blood. These regions are places of greatest vulnerability. It is believed that, in particular, they suffer most severely from " fatigue poisons ", and from drugs and chemical substances of all sorts, including such anæsthetics as chloroform and ether.

(6) THE GENERAL SCHEME ON WHICH THE NERVOUS SYSTEM IS CONSTRUCTED

Although apparently so complicated, the plan of construction of the nervous system is simple; it consists of ingoing neurons, outgoing neurons and a vast number of neurons which connect these (inter-nuncial or commissural neurons). In Fig. 7 let us begin with the nerve-cells C_1 C_2 and C_3, which are situated in the spinal cord. They are the cells of origin of nerve-fibres (E. N.) which descend as the motor nerves of muscles. The neuron (E. N.) is an efferent neuron. All the cells of the C order are found either in the spinal cord or in its upward extension, the Bulb (medulla oblongata.) For short we call this series of nerve-cells the central nervous axis, and regard it as the lowest functional realm.

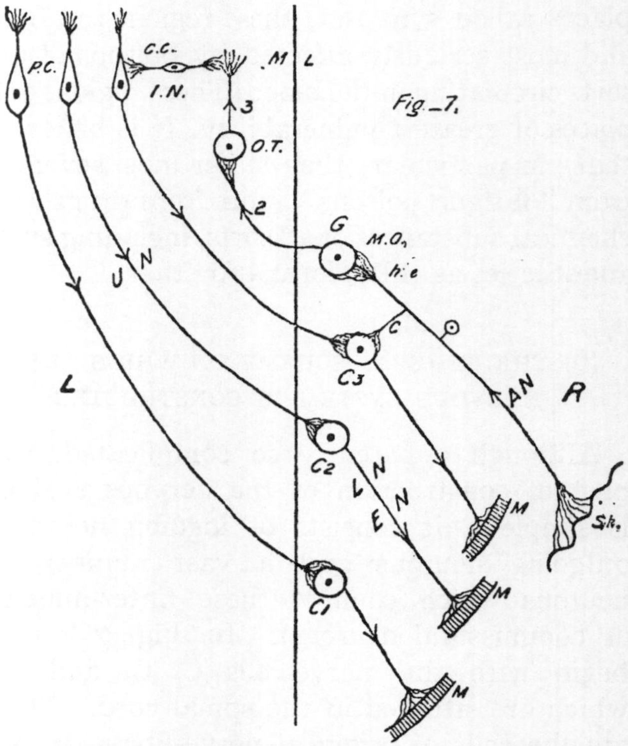

Diagram showing crossed relationships of upper neurons (N.U.) and lower neurons (L.N.).

C_1 C_2 and C_3 motor-centres in spinal cord, cells of origin for efferent neurons, E.N. These also are lower neurons, L.N. for M the muscles. P.C. pyramidal cells of grey matter of brain. C.C. cortex cerebri giving origin to upper neurons, U.N.

Sk. skin in which arises afferent neuron, A.N. which ends over a "sensory" cell, G. in medulla oblongata. A second neuron arising in G crosses mid-line (M.L.) and ends over cell of Optic Thalamus (O.T.) The third upward neuron (3) terminates in grey matter of brain (sensory centre). Sensory centres are linked to motor (P.C.) by inter-nuncial neurons I.N.

Referring again to Fig. 7, we notice that the cells of the C order are related to neurons which descend on them from the grey matter of the brain (cortex cerebri). The cells of origin of these cerebral neurons are called "pyramidal cells", and they are related to the cells of the C order by a crossed relationship (decussation).

Thus, the left side of the brain governs the muscles on the right side of the body and vice versa. The cerebral fibres are often called the Upper Neurons (U.N.), and the spinal and Bulbar, the Lower Neurons (L.N.).

This crossed relationship explains why when a person gets an injury or serious internal bleeding on the left side of the brain, the muscles on the right side are paralyzed.

The same crossed relationship subsists in regard to the sensory fibres. These afferent fibres, which arise in the skin of the right side of the body, pass up the spinal cord to end synaptically over cells in the medulla oblongata. Here a second neuron has its origin in the cell G, whose fibre crosses mid-line and ascends towards the left side of the brain. This second ascending neuron does not, however, go all the way to the cortex, but has a cell-station (synapsis) in a region known to anatomists as the Optic

Thalamus. This is one of the masses of nerve-cells called " Basal ganglia ", and here the third afferent neuron takes its origin.

There are, then, two interruptions (synapses) on the course of the afferent path from the surface of the body to the grey matter of the brain. Thus the left side of the brain receives sensory impressions from the right side of the body, which is the side we have seen it controls motorially.

Fig. 7 is useful in one more respect, for it shows how a reflex arc is related to the afferent and efferent neurons we have just been considering. From the afferent neuron, A. N., comes off the collateral *c*, which by ending synaptically over C_3 establishes a skin-to-muscle reflex arc. The headward extension (*h*, *e*) is the physical basis for the sensation which may be aroused at the time at which reflex action is taking place over the arc through C_3 as a centre.

Reflex action will be discussed in Chapter IV.

CHAPTER III

THE NATURE OF THE NERVE-IMPULSE

All living protoplasm possesses affectability,[1] the power or property of responding to a stimulus. For our present purpose we may define the "stimulus" as, that agent or agency which elicits a response from the living matter. The three concepts, stimulus, affectability and response are thus causally linked, and one of them has no meaning apart from the other two.

A living muscle in virtue of its affectability on receiving a stimulus—electric shock, a blow, a chemical irritant—responds by a twitch or "contraction", a shortening. Similarly a nerve, by reason of its affectability on receiving a stimulus, conveys a nerve-impulse.

If we decapitate a frog and remove from its leg the gastrocnemius muscle with a

[1] This property is generally called irritability, but since this term has a certain popular meaning, the more exclusive term is to be preferred.

length of nerve (sciatic) attached to it, both the nerve and the muscle, if kept in a cool, moist atmosphere, will live for many hours. If we send a momentary electric shock through the far end of the nerve, we notice that the muscle at the other end shortens for an instant and then elongates, in other words twitches.

If we give two stimuli to the far end of the nerve, the muscle will twitch twice. Evidently the stimulus to the end of the nerve has caused something to descend the nerve and throw the muscle into activity. This " something " we call the nerve-impulse. But all nerves do not innervate muscles; if we stimulate the nerve to a blood-vessel (arteriole) it will become narrower; if the nerve to a gland, the gland will secrete ; if to the iris, the pupil will be dilated, and so on.

All we are concerned with at present is that if we stimulate an efferent nerve, and something happens in the tissue to which that nerve is distributed, something must have travelled from the point of stimulation to the periphery, and that " something " is the nerve-impulse. The stimulation starts a state of excitation which travels down the nerve and becomes the stimulus for the muscle to contract, the vessel to constrict, the gland to secrete or the pupil to dilate. Because such a state of excitation can travel down the nerve we speak of the nerve possessing the property of conductivity.

This property of conductivity—the power of transmitting a molecular disturbance—is possessed in some degree by all living matter, most obviously by muscle. If we chill a long muscle, we can actually *see* the state of contraction passing over it from one end to the other. The nerve-fibre however has been specialized to *conduct;* in fact, we know of no other function or property it has than that of conducting impulses. A nerve is a living linear conductor of impulses and of nothing else. Neural conductivity is to be distinguished both from thermal and electrical.

This conductivity can be mechanically abolished by a ligature drawn sufficiently tightly around the nerve. Any kind of pressure, if powerful enough, will interfere with the passage of the impulses. Thus, the pressure of a crutch in the arm-pit will paralyze certain muscles of the arm, because it cuts off nerve-impulses in the nerve which innervates those muscles.

By freezing a nerve we can abolish its conductivity, partially or entirely, for this does not injure the fibres as pressure does.

This method as applied to sensory nerves of the gum is sometimes used by dentists, who freeze the gum before they pull out a tooth. It is known as local anæsthesia.

In yet another way we can abolish the conductivity of a nerve, namely by applying to it—and especially to its terminations—various drugs or chemical substances such as ether, chloroform, and ethyl chloride. Such substances are called local anæsthetics, or more specifically analgesics (abolishers of pain).

The only evidence we have, then, of the passage of a nerve-impulse is some activity at the periphery in the case of efferent nerves and of some modification of consciousness in the case of afferent.

There is, luckily, an objective accompaniment of the passage of the nerve-impulse in an electrical disturbance which is propagated along the nerve exactly as is the nerve-impulse itself. If we cut off the muscle from the end of the nerve, and place the nerve over the " lead-off " electrodes of a galvanometer (an instrument which records electric currents even when feeble and brief) then, on stimulating the far end of the nerve, a current is found to pass through the galvanometer. This electric disturbance is the outward and visible sign of the passing of a nerve-impulse, and, as it happens, is a conveniently measurable one. Very fortunately it can be photographed. If a series of stimuli are given to the nerve, a corresponding series of electric responses at the same rhythm appears in the galvanometer. The experiment can be varied in the manner designed by the late Professor A. D. Waller thus :—

The stimulations can be given in the middle of a length of nerve which has still its muscle at one end and is in contact with the galvanometer at the other.

At each stimulus, one obtains simultaneously a muscular twitch and a galvanometric deflection, clearly showing that muscle and the galvanometer are both actuated by the same thing—the nerve-impulse. Incidentally it shows that an efferent nerve can conduct equally well in both directions, a phenomenon sometimes called " the law of double conduction ". This " Law " is just as true of afferent nerves.

The electric disturbance in a nerve is not

an isolated phenomenon ; all protoplasm in activity gives rise to electric current ; muscle and the heart notably do so. It would appear that just as muscle cannot contract without producing heat and electric current, so nerve cannot conduct without also producing heat and electric current, but the heat produced is very small.

The next point we should notice in regard to the nerve-impulse is that no matter by what different kinds of stimulus it has been started, it is always of the same kind. The muscle of a nerve-muscle preparation will twitch whether the nerve has been stimulated electrically, chemically, thermally or mechanically.

The galvanometer always shows an electric current whether the nerve is faradized, galvanized, heated, pinched or has salt put on it.

Applying this to the living body, we do not believe that there is any difference between nerve-impulses whether they are sensory or whether they excite muscles, glands or blood-vessels. This was not, however, the view once held ; quite the contrary. It was once supposed that all these impulses were different the one from the other ; but all recent evidence points to nerve-impulses being identical when travelling in the nerves; the result or action at the periphery depends entirely on the kind of organ or tissue on which the nerve ends.

In no matter how many different ways we stimulate a sensory nerve, we always have the same sensation as the result.[1] It has been discovered experimentally that mechanical, chemical or electrical stimulations of the nerve of taste (chorda tympani) all produce the sensation of the same taste.

An exactly similar state of matters is true of the retina which is a complicated nerve-net; both mechanical and electrical stimulations of it give rise to the sensation of light. Again in the case of the ear, not only sound-waves but pressure on the nerve of hearing will give rise to sounds. A plug of wax pressing on the membrane of the drum of the ear can give rise to a ringing sound.

A too high pressure of blood in the neighbourhood of the auditory nerve will give rise to sounds—so-called "subjective" sounds.

If in any one sensory nerve the kind of stimulation does not determine the kind of sensation, then the kind of sensation must

[1] This was originally called the Law of "specific nerve energy".

depend on that particular part of the brain in which the nerve ends. In other words, as in efferent nerves the specificity resides in the peripheral organs, so in afferent nerves it resides in the central locations, the sensory centres in the brain.

The fact of the non-specificity of nerve-impulses is made practical use of by the surgeon in cases of "nerve-crossing". The following is an example: it sometimes happens that the nerve for the muscles of expression (the seventh cranial) is cut accidentally, and for some reason the upper end does not regenerate so far as the muscles of the face. The surgeon can sometimes cause certain fibres of the spinal accessory nerve (ninth cranial) to cross over into the degenerated facial nerve. The spinal accessory supplies the long muscle which turns the head to right or left as well as the muscle which raises the shoulder. In the operation, the entire nerve was not cut across (which would have paralyzed these two great muscles), but only some of its fibres were divided so that the central ends of these cut fibres were caused to cross over into the peripheral end of the facial nerve.

The functional result of this was that

when the man smiled he also had always to shrug the shoulder on the side of the operated nerve.

THE RATE OF PROPAGATION OF THE NERVE-IMPULSE

If the nerve-impulse is a real state of excitement travelling along a nerve, its velocity should be capable of being ascertained.

This was first calculated in the motor nerves of the frog and found to be about 28 metres a second. This was first calculated by the eminent German mathematician and physiologist, Hermann Helmholtz at Königsberg. In 1835 Johannes Müller, another German physiologist, had unfortunately predicted that the speed of "nervous action" was incalculably rapid. He wrote: "We shall probably never attain the power of measuring the velocity of nervous action, for we have not the opportunity of comparing its propagation through immense spaces, as we have in the case of light".

Fifteen years afterwards, Helmholtz ascertained that the velocity was not only calculable, but not by any means excessively great. Helmholtz ascertained the rate of the impulse in the intact nerve of man where he found it about 120 metres a second. From very accurate observations in 1912 by an electrical method, Piper of Kiel found the rate in human nerves to be 123 metres a second.

The rate in afferent is the same as in efferent fibres. All workers are agreed that the strength of the stimulus does not affect the velocity; but that the temperature of the nerve has a distinct influence on it.

The rate of the propagation of the impulses is by no means the same throughout all classes of animals.

Carlson, the American physiologist, has investigated it in several types; his results are given in the following table—

Animal	*Rate in metres per second at 17°C (air temp.)*
Man	120
Frog	28
Snake	14
Lobster	12
Hag-fish	4.5
King-crab (Limulus)	3.25
Octopus	2.00
Slug (Limax)	1.25
Heart plexus of Limulus	0.4

In other words, the more lowly the animal in the zoological scale, the slower is the rate of its neural conduction, which is rather what one would have expected.

NERVE-FIBRES AND FATIGUE

The last subject we shall investigate is the alleged impossibility of fatiguing a nerve. By "fatigue" we mean relative functional incapacity due to previous activity which can be recovered from, whereas by exhaustion we mean a state which cannot be recovered from. In physiological fatigue no permanent damage is done; in exhaustion it is.

By no known experimental method can we discover the presence of fatigue in nerve-fibres; that is to say, nerve-fibres stimulated electrically for many hours still gave galvanometric evidence of the passage of nerve-impulses. As the late Dr Waller said: "You will be tired before the nerve will". This indefatigability of nerves is true of nerves both *in situ* and excised—and excised nerve, if kept in saline solution, will remain alive for several days. In this respect the nerve-fibre resembles a telephone wire which shows no fatigue even when the speakers at each end and the people in the exchange may be all exhausted.

The nerves are true conductors only, and show no diminution in this capacity however long they may have been employed.

Nerves require oxygen in order to remain in a state of functional integrity. We know of no unassailable fact to indicate that they have anything but the feeblest chemical activity.

Professor A. V. Hill, F.R.S., by an extremely delicate method, has detected a slight amount of heat during the activity of nerve-fibre.

Within the last few years a considerable amount of information regarding the behaviour of the impulses travelling in the nerves has been acquired. These researches have been carried out by Dr E. D. Adrian, F.R.S., and his co-workers at Cambridge.

The investigation has been made possible by employing a method involving the use of the thermionic valve and a capillary electrometer whereby the action-currents of nerve are enormously amplified and then photographed.

Some notion of the sensitiveness of the apparatus may be had when we are told that it can detect a charge of potential amounting to 0.01 millivolts lasting only for the one-thousandth of a second.

Dr. Adrian has demonstrated what we previously only believed, namely, that during life, streams or series of impulses are continually ascending and descending the living nerve-fibres. The sensory nerves of muscle were those first studied. Dr Adrian wished, if possible, to record the impulses ascending a single afferent nerve in order, of course, not to have the record complicated by the fusion of currents-of-action due to numbers of neighbouring fibres.

A muscle was used, because the sensory organs of muscle so familiar to microscopists are relatively large, and in a small muscle are comparatively few.

Selecting a very small muscle from the frog, with its nerve intact, Dr Adrian fastened the muscle securely and allowed a hanging weight to act as its stimulus. The tiny nerve contained only from 12 to 25 fibres, the most of which were motor. The conditions desired seem to be realized as nearly as possible —to have an afferent nerve stimulated in the natural way and its resultant impulses visibly recorded. So small a weight as two grammes was used at first, and allowed to act for ten seconds before the photograph was taken. When this was done, Dr Adrian obtained a record of a series of action-currents ascending the nerve at a rhythm of from 22 to 25 a second. The number of impulses per second (frequency) was found to be somewhat increased as the magnitude of the stimulus (weight) was increased thus—in one experiment, with a weight of $\frac{1}{4}$ gramme, the frequency was 21, with $\frac{1}{2}$ a gramme, 27, and with one gramme, 33 a second.

Increase of the magnitude of the stimulus while it increased the rate of the rhythm of the responses did *not* increase their ampitude. Thus an eight-fold increase in the weight gave no increase in the magnitude of the impulses.

This is a special case of the " all or nothing " law, as it has been picturesquely called.

If the nerve-fibre responds at all, it responds to its utmost (maximally). The heart muscle is the typical example of this maximal response to stimuli of all intensities. The fact that when the stimulus is constant (a given weight) the nerve impulses are rhythmic, must be due to some property of the end-organs and not of the nerve itself. For it has long been known that a constant stimulus to a nerve-fibre produces one initial response and not a series of responses.

In other words, the power to transform the constant stimulus into the *series* of nerve-impulses must be a property of the sensory end-organs of the muscle. What the nature of this property is must be a problem for future research.

Even when no weight at all was acting on the muscle, that is when the muscle was in complete physiological rest, impulses at 3 to 8 a second were still ascending the nerve-fibres.

Dr Adrian has also investigated the optic nerve by the same apparatus. Here of course the electrometer is connected to the optic nerve, and the retina of the eye is stimulated by flashes of light. Distinct evidence was obtained that a single flash on the retina produced rhythmic impulses in the optic nerve, but, for certain reasons, the frequency of these could not be accurately computed.

The motor nerves of muscle have been investigated by the same method of photography, and the conclusion come to that the frequency of impulses in the efferent nerves is of the order of 50 to 70 a second. This is now thought to "represent the proper rhythm of the motor spinal neurons".

CHAPTER IV

REFLEX ACTION

Reflex action is the type of action within the central nervous system.

A reflex action is one which, involving the central nervous system, is not volitional and not automatic. The beat of the heart is automatic in that it can go on after all nerves are cut and when that organ is removed from the body.[1] Frequent as volitional action is, it is probably not so common as is reflex, for certain reflexes such as those which maintain the tone of skeletal muscles never cease day or night.

Reflex action had better be studied in a concrete case. If we decapitate a frog, and thus at " one fell swoop " abolish its volition and all its consciousness by destroying its brain, the spinal cord and the rest of the body will live for many hours.

[1]The heart of the warm-blooded animal, if supplied with blood, will beat for some hours outside the body; the heart of a cold-blooded animal will beat for some days even without blood.

If now we hang up this unconscious, headless " preparation " on a hook, it will assume under gravity a perfectly limp, vertical position. It appears to be dead, for it is motionless; but if we were to open its chest we should find the heart still beating and the blood circulating, therefore it is still alive.

If, after a little while, we stroke one of the flanks, we shall find that certain muscles under the skin begin to twitch, but they stop the moment we cease the stimulation.

We can make this phenomenon more spectacular by placing on the flank a small piece of blotting-paper steeped in weak acid. Nothing seems to be happening for a second or two, when a twitching is seen in some of the toes on the same side of the body. In an instant more, the leg of that side is lifted up, and the foot swiftly brought to the place where the irritant paper is sticking. So precisely is this usually accomplished and the paper flicked off so accurately, that one cannot rid oneself of the impression that it is being done voluntarily by a fully conscious animal.

This action we call a " reflex action "—a muscular reflex. But the muscle was not directly stimulated ; it was the *skin* that was stimulated (*Sk* in Fig. 8) ; it is as though something had ascended from the skin at

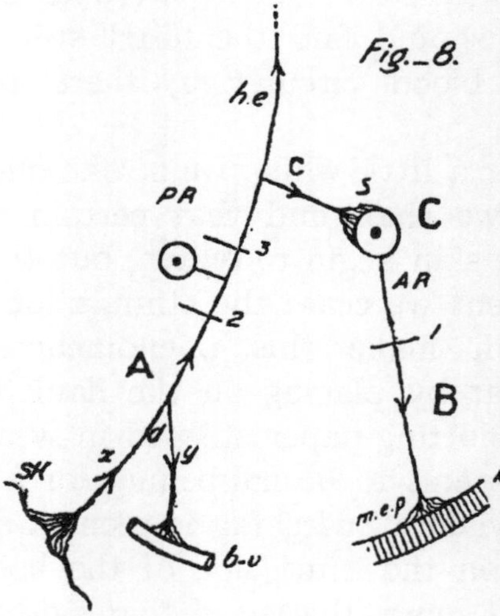

Diagram of a simple Reflex Nerve-Arc.

Sk **the skin ; A, afferent neuron with headward extension *h.e.* and collateral, *c*, ending in synapse S over cell, C, of a reflex centre.**
B, efferent neuron to muscle *m*, *m.e.p.* motor end-plate.
***d*, place of division of axon. *b.v.*, blood-vessel in skin.**
A is a nerve-fibre in the posterior root.
B is a nerve-fibre from the anterior root.
1, 2 and 3 are sites of sections.

the periphery to the spinal cord and been sent back, *reflected*, to the periphery again, this time not to the skin, but to the muscles (*m*, Fig. 8); the spinal cord has acted *like* a reflector (*s*,C, Fig. 8).

We may learn a good deal from this brainless frog. First, that this raising of the leg is definitely in response to the stimulation of the skin, and is not spontaneous, for a decapitated frog will otherwise hang by its neck until it becomes a mummy. It will never make one spontaneous effort to escape.

It is in fact a mindless automaton, although an animal organism; it has no spontaneity nor initiative; it would hang on the hook for ever. It moves only in response to the stimulation of the skin, it is these movements we call "reflexes"; the frog is, therefore, now only a reflex mechanism. But as nothing was done to it except to cut off its head, its spinal cord must have been a reflex mechanism before; and so indeed it was; but in the head was the brain, which could in some way influence, control, augment or interfere with the reflex mechanisms placed lower down in the central nervous system. No creature with a spark of consciousness left in it would thus hang motionless until it dried up without making some efforts to escape.

The machine-like response to the stimulation of its skin is remarkable; as often as you place the acid paper on its flank will its toes be brought up towards that spot; only fatigue of the spinal cord makes it fail.

Finally, if we destroy the spinal cord by "pithing" it, all reflexes are completely and permanently abolished.

Instead of decapitating the frog, which allows of some loss of blood, we may "pith" the brain by simply forcing a wooden match into the inside of the skull and leaving it there. By this method practically no blood is lost, but the frog is rendered perfectly unconscious.

Having assured ourselves that there are no signs of consciousness in the headless or brain-pithed frog, how shall we describe its act in flicking the paper off its side? For if consciousness has gone, that means that sensation and volition, both modes of consciousness, have gone also. It simply means that however "purposeful" the action looks, it is *not* purposeful, if that implies due to, or accompanied by, consciousness.

We can bring out an action apparently more purposeful still; for if we apply to the left flank a stronger irritant in the form of a bit of paper steeped in stronger acid, and at the same time hold down the left foot, then after a short interval, the leg of the *opposite* side will be brought over and attempt to flick off the paper. An onlooker who did not know that the frog had had its brain pithed, would at once conclude it did it " on purpose". It looks like sensation, will and intelligence, while it is nothing of the sort.

We must sharply distinguish the automatic action from the reflex; although each can proceed in the complete absence of consciousness. The term "automatic" is purely descriptive; it indicates no theory; it merely states that something is going on "of itself" (*autos* self, and *mao,* I move). The heart-beat is the typical example of an automatic action. The term asserts nothing except that the activity is going on without apparent stimulus or encouragement from without. By reflex action we mean at least that it involves the nervous system (which some automatic actions do not), and does *not* go on of itself (spontaneously), but, on the contrary, always in response to a stimulus.

A reflex action, therefore, is some activity at the periphery in consequence of some stimulation at the periphery. In the case of the decapitated frog, the skin was the peripheral spot stimulated, and the muscle the peripheral organ activated,. More technically, we could define a reflex action as the activity of an effector in consequence of the previous activity of a receptor.

Fig. 8 shows all these points. *Sk* is the skin, *m* the muscle, A the receptor, B the effector. C is the centre and *c* a collateral having its synapsis, *s*, over C.

All reflex actions are not entirely outside the conscious sphere as we shall presently see ; and this gives us the first basis of classification of these actions, namely into lower and higher.

By a " low " reflex we mean one which is neither caused by a conscious state nor involved in one. It is carried out entirely outside or below the conscious realm.

Such reflexes are called " Excito-motor ". A typical, lower, excito-motor reflex has therefore, three characteristics as follow—

1. It is not produced by a conscious factor :
2. It does not arouse or involve consciousness :
3. It cannot be voluntarily restrained (inhibited).

Evidently the reflexes in the decapitated frog are excito-motor, as they conform to all of these conditions.

If we refer to Fig. 8 we see there portrayed the minimal number of anatomical structures required for a reflex action; namely, one afferent neuron A, and one efferent neuron B. This path from the periphery through a centre, and back to the periphery again, is called a "reflex nerve-arc". It is a skin-to-muscle-arc.

This was the term given to it about 1832 by the English physiologist and clincian, Dr Marshall Hall (1790-1857).

In this, the simplest of all arcs, only two neurons therefore are involved. The "centre" is the nerve-cell trophic for the efferent neuron (C, Fig. 8). No arc can be simpler than this: a collateral carries the impulses from A to B. The collateral ends in a brush of filaments over the cell-body C.

But the actual varieties of the excito-motor reflex are very many. Thus, instead of in the skin, the stimuli may arise in any of the mucous membranes from the nose to the depths of the lung or from the mouth to the rectum.

Similarly, instead of a body-muscle as an

effector, we may have the muscle of heart, or blood-vessel, or of intestine, bladder, bronchial tube, iris, or reproductive organ.

The anatomical types are many, the physiological principle is the same in all these lowly reflexes.

In the intact human being such reflexes as are carried out in sleep, which do not appeal to consciousness and cannot be inhibited by the will, are excito-motor. In the injured human being, excito-motor reflexes are seen in the serious disease, paraplegia, which is paralysis of the legs owing to conduction being interrupted in the spinal cord. Usually it is the result of an accident in which the cord is severed in the back (" back broken "). The legs are " paralyzed " because impulses of voluntary (cerebral) origin cannot reach the centres of the nerves which supply them, the legs " feel nothing " (are anæsthetic) because the sensory tracts of the cord are similarly interrupted.

Now whereas the patient is completely unable to move his legs, of which he has no knowledge except that of sight, a very slight tickling on the soles of the feet will cause powerful jerking movements of the legs and toes. These are clearly excito-motor reflexes from the soles of the feet to the muscles of the toes, the arcs being from the skin to these muscles.

The evacuations of the bowel and the bladder in these unfortunate patients are carried out in a wholly reflex manner. There are similar reflexes involving the reproductive organs. In the nature of the case, the person cannot have control over any of these happenings. The lower portion of his spinal cord has now an independent existence. The lower portion of the cord is no longer part of a person, but a series of independent reflex centres.

The " person ", through a purely mechanical accident, has now no longer any control over or knowledge of a portion of his own body. This portion exhibits the primitive reflex character of a segmented animal.

A useful working classification of reflexes is to name them according to the effectors utilized. Thus the Excito-motor reflexes would be—

Excito-muscular, excito-vascular, excito-glandular and excito-metabolic, according as the effectors, respectively, are the muscles, the heart and blood-vessels, the glands, and the tissues exclusive of these.

A good example of an *excito-muscular* reflex is the last stage of swallowing solid food. This is the well-known stage when the morsel is "beyond recall". The physiological reason of that is, it is beyond the reach of voluntary inhibition. This stage can go on during unconsciousness, as when an unconscious person swallows the stomach-pump. This happens when that instrument is passed into the stomach of a person "dead" drunk. He cannot carry out the first or voluntary stage of swallowing, but the last stage is carried out reflexly or independently of the intoxicated person's knowledge or sensations.

Swallowing depends on the integrity of a reflex nerve-arc.

This reflex swallowing conforms, then, to the three criteria of excito-motor reflexes; for it is not due to consciousness, it is not an appeal to consciousness, and it cannot be inhibited by the will.

Hiccough is another example of an *excito-muscular* reflex action; the diaphragm is caused to contract in a jerky fashion owing to some irritation, usually to the mucous membrane of the stomach. This reflex cannot really be inhibited by the will, and it can proceed in an unconscious person.

Vomiting is another *excito-muscular* reflex; it is carried out jointly by abdominal muscles and the muscles of the stomach itself. The nausea that precedes it is no part of the reflex action. It certainly can go on in the unconscious person, as every surgeon knows; and unfortunately it cannot be inhibited by the will.

The heart-muscle is easily accessible to reflex influences, and these are chiefly met with in abnormal states of the internal organs. The same is true of the muscle of the blood-vessels; certain flushings of the skin are expressions of reflex irritation from internal organs.

Excito-glandular: in some forms of indigestion, the saliva flows from the mouth, and this is especially so just before vomiting takes place. Here the irritated mucous membrane of the stomach is the source of the reflex salivation. This salivation is quite outside the sphere of voluntary control.

The *excito-metabolic* group of reflexes is the most indefinite of all. By "metabolic" is meant the chemical side of tissue activity.

We have reason to believe that reflex influences are continually and unconsciously descending from the nervous system upon all tissues—muscles, glands, and blood-vessels—keeping these in a state of proper chemical (metabolic) "tone". Such nerves used to be called "trophic".

The next and very large group of reflex actions is that called the *Sensori-motor*. Here a sensation accompanies the action, but it is a concomitant occurrence, and not the cause of the reflex.

As previously, a concrete example had better be taken. We all know that when a small piece of grit gets into the eye, the eye begins to "water". In reality, the foreign body has lodged between the cornea and the eyelid, and so irritated these surfaces that impulses are sent up to the central nervous system, whence other impulses are sent down to the tear (lachrymal) gland in the orbit. This gland pours out its watery secretion to wash away the offending particle.

There must be a centre governing or presiding over the outflow of the tears which is roused to action by a receptor and in turn activates an effector. There is, in other words, a reflex nerve-arc which includes a centre; and the fact that the grit causes discomfort or pain is not any necessary factor in the performance of the reflex action.

That sensation is aroused is due to the fact that there is a headward extension (*h. e.*) of the afferent neuron A (Fig. 8) which conveys impulses to the sensory portion of the cortex cerebri. This reflex is evidently sensori-glandular,[1] but it is not the existence of the sensation that excites the reflex. The gland will secrete even in a person whose consciousness has been abolished by an anæsthetic. The sensation is present, but not casually present; it is what Huxley called an "epiphenomenon". It need scarcely be pointed out that the will has no power whatever over this flow of tears; as a reflex it cannot be voluntarily inhibited.

For another example of a sensori-motor reflex we may take the case of the dentist and his attentions to our teeth and gums. We know that it is not long before the saliva begins to flow so freely that it requires to be drained away or continually mopped up. It is a sensori-glandular reflex.

The reflexes of the eye are very important. Most people know that a bright light makes the pupil contract. We can see in a mirror the pupil contracting; or another person can

[1] In Fig. 8, a muscle is represented as the effector; but the scheme is exactly the same when the efferent neuron (B) ends on a gland or a blood-vessel.

observe it and tell us of it, but we are totally unaware of the presence and behaviour of our iris or its reflexes. We cannot voluntarily contract or dilate the pupil.

This reflex, known as the pupillary or " light reflex ", is utilized by the anæsthetist to inform him of the depth of what is called " surgical anæsthesia ". The surgeon wishes to abolish from his patients not only pain, but also all musculo-motor reflexes which, if not so got rid of, would seriously interfere with the niceties of his operation. It is perfectly clear that if the patient could struggle all the time that the surgeon was carrying out the delicate procedures of modern surgical technique, the surgeon would be very greatly hampered. A return to the undesirable speed of the bad, old, pre-chloroform days would be rendered necessary. Only in the earlier stages of chloroform anæsthesia is the pupillary reflex obtained, so the anæsthetist uses the moment of the disappearance of the " light reflex " (as, for short, he calls the reflex pupillo-constriction) to indicate the moment when the surgeon may begin to cut the skin. For when the chloroform has so raised the resistance to the passage of impulses over the centre for the light reflex that stimulation of the retina by light fails to arouse to activity the effectors of the iris, the surgeon is sure that the chloroform will have raised the resistance in those synapses in the cerebrum which are related to the development of sensation and pain. Pain being abolished, the surgeon may safely begin.

We classify the sensori-motor reflexes exactly as we have the excito-motor, namely, into sensori-muscular, sensori-vascular, sensori-glandular, and sensori-metabolic.

Sensori-muscular. This is a very large group ; for the effectors here include skeletal muscles, the heart, and the muscles of the abdominal viscera, the so-called smooth or involuntary muscle.

The inevitable jerk we give when a pin is stuck into us is a sensori-muscular reflex ; coughing from irritation in the lungs is another example ; sneezing from a bright light is a third ; the blinking of the eyelids at a threatened blow is a fourth.

Sensori-vascular. These reflexes are also very numerous. When a cold draught on the skin makes its blood-vessels blanch (contract) we have a sensori-vascular reflex. When, conversely, heat makes them dilate, we have reflex flushing (vaso-dilatation).

Sensori-glandular. Perspiration through the action of heat is such a reflex. It is not due to the heat acting directly on the glands in the skin, but to the heat stimulating the nerve-endings. For if the (sciatic) nerve in one leg of a cat is cut, and the animal placed in a warm box, it will perspire on the three pads supplied by the intact nerves, but not on the fourth pad, which is equally exposed to the heat.

The flow of saliva in consequence of some taste in the mouth is another example of a sensori-glandular reflex.

Reflexes accompanied by pain. As examples of these reflexes we have the contortions and violent muscular efforts due to severe pain. A large number of the muscular reflexes occur in the muscles of the intestines and in the ducts of the abdominal viscera.

" Colic " itself is often a reflex spasm of the muscular coats of the stomach or intestine produced by some kind of irritation to the mucous membrane—indigestible food, etc. The passage of a calculus in the bile-duct or in the duct of the kidney which may be extremely painful can give rise to such wide-spread reflexes as flushing, perspiration, alteration in the rhythm and force of the heart, and in vomiting. The vomiting centre which is in the medulla oblongata is particularly accessible to afferent impulses coming in over a large number of receptors.

Painful reflexes, owing to the violence of their action, are peculiarly liable to spread and irradiate throughout the central nervous axis.

Some allusion must be made to the important subject of Referred Sensation and Referred Pain, a species of irradiation. It is familiar to many people that in disease of the liver, for instance, there is a pain behind the right shoulder blade, in heart disease in the left arm, and in indigestion behind the breast-bone—

> " It's that confounded cucumber
> I've eat and can't digest."
> —*Ingoldsby Legends.*

These sensations or pains, as the case may be, are referred or transferred from the seat of the irritation to a place where there is no disease at all. A patch of skin has had referred to it a pain of which it is not the seat or origin.

This curious condition will be made clear from a study of Fig. 9, which is a scheme of the relations of the neurons involved. L_1 is the liver or other internal organ, and L the afferent neuron arising in the liver and passing upwards into the spinal cord, somewhere from the headward extension of the neuron (h_1e_1) a collateral C_1 enters the central grey matter of the spinal cord (G.M.C). In this region, the collateral (C) of an afferent

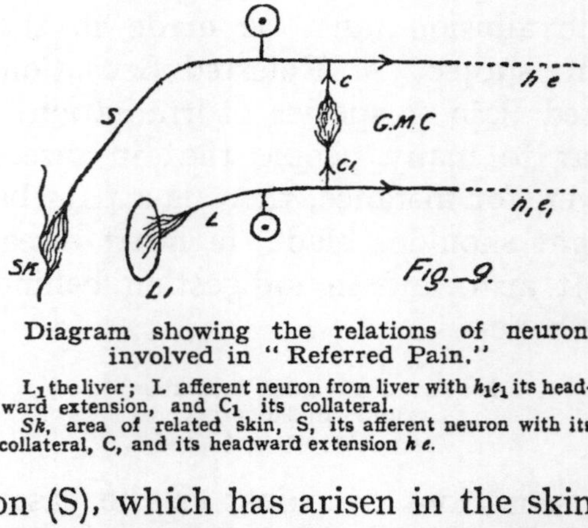

Diagram showing the relations of neurons involved in "Referred Pain."

L_1 the liver; L afferent neuron from liver with h_1e_1 its headward extension, and C_1 its collateral.
Sk, area of related skin, S, its afferent neuron with its collateral, C, and its headward extension *h e*.

neuron (S), which has arisen in the skin (*Sk*) also enters the spinal grey matter, and here, for some reason not fully understood, the impulses passing over C_1 become transferred to C. The impulses passing over L ought normally to be of an order quite subconscious, but when L_1 is the seat of disease, the impulses in L are evidently so violent that they ascend in the headward extension, giving rise to the pain, and they overflow in the collateral (C_1) on to the related collateral (C). But the impulses being transferred to S on reaching a sensory centre by the headward extension (*he.*) give rise to a sensation *as though* the area of skin (*Sk*) had itself been stimulated. Thus the irritation which began in the liver is transferred to a neuron from the skin, and the mind is constrained to refer the seat of that irritation to the skin over the right shoulder. The neuron from the liver and the neuron from the skin enter the same region of the cord, and here the transference takes place.

It will readily be seen how the knowledge of the relationship of the visible surface of the body to some invisible internal organ may be of value to the medical man, because he can tell which internal organ is at fault by ascertaining which particular region of skin is experiencing the sensation or the pain.

Referred sensations may be of the nature of itchings, burnings, or stabbings. In some cases they are momentary annoyances, in others constant discomforts. The spot of skin which is the seat of the referred sensation may actually be quite tender or painful to touch.

The area of skin to which pains are referred need not necessarily be over the internal seat of the irritation. Thus, many headaches are due to disorder in the stomach. in which case the reference is to the head, a part of the body tolerably remote from the organ primarily affected.

Sensori-metabolic: here we have a group of effects upon tissues carried out reflexly —the stimulus involving sensation. The stimulant influence of light is a case in point; all animals are in better condition when in well-lighted places than in the contrary. Cows in well-lighted byres give richer milk than those in gloomy sheds.

CHAPTER V

THE HIGHER REFLEX ACTIONS

In the sensori-motor reflex we saw that on the anatomical side the element of consciousness was introduced by the fact that a headward extension of the afferent limb of the reflex arc entered the cerebral cortex or region of consciousness (*h.e.* in Figs. 7 and 8).

On the psychic side this extension involves the presence of a sensation not causally but only as an "epi-phenomenon", as Huxley phrased it. But the long or cerebral arc having been laid down, the cortex has been brought into the reflex scheme, and in the psycho-motor reflexes which we are about to study the cerebral portion of the arc is an integral portion of the neural mechanism.

The emotion or idea, as the case may be, which is the psychic factor in the reflex, is a causal antecedent. As before, a specific example will be best.

Blushing is perhaps one of the most familiar of vascular actions. The centre involved is clearly the vaso-motor centre in the Bulb, the centre devoted to maintaining a moderate degree of tone in the arterioles.

The circular muscle of these small arteries is always tending to open out, but the continual innervation keeps the circular muscle moderately contracted.

Now the " seat " of the emotion is not in the Bulb but in the cortex cerebri, from which impulses descend on to the vaso-motor centre, lessening its tone (inhibiting it) so that it innervates the arterioles less intensely, so that they dilate.

The existence of emotion is, therefore, *causal* in this case: a cerebral state has influenced the tone of a lower centre. This blushing is an activity involving consciousness not merely as an accessory phenomenon, which we have seen in sensori-motor reflexes, but as the cause itself; such a reflex is a psycho-motor one.

Blushing is reflex because it is neither an automatic nor a voluntary act, and it is brought about through a centre situated below the region of consciousness.

It is notoriously not a voluntary act;

this was noticed long ago by Seneca, who said: " The Roman players hang down their heads, fix their eyes on the ground, and keep them lowered; but are unable to blush in acting shame ".

What the will cannot do, emotion often can. Just as blushing cannot be produced by the will, neither can it be restrained thereby. Sometimes it would be convenient for the shy or guilty person if it could be voluntarily inhibited, but it cannot be.

We may classify the Emotio-motor reflexes on the same basis as the other types according as muscles, heart, blood-vessels or glands are effectors.

Where skeletal muscle is involved, we have such phenomena as trembling from rage or terror; sighing, " holding the breath from fear ", and a large number of other interferences with the respiratory rhythm. The dog on meeting his enemy bristles up, here the muscles involved are those of the hairs. Other examples are such reflexes as the pupil dilated from fear, and all those alterations of the tone of the muscles of the digestive tube, or of the urinary bladder, or of the reproductive organs.

Various people react differently to these

emotions; in some, the peristalsis[1] of the intestine is so much increased that they suffer from diarrhœa, in others the peristalsis is quelled and they have constipation.

The emotional reflexes involving the blood-vessels are perhaps the most familiar to the majority of people. The increased or disturbed action of the heart under the influence of emotion has been observed from time immemorial.

The heart is so susceptible to reflexes accompanying the "softer" emotions, that the word "heart" has come to be a synonym for these emotions themselves as is testified to daily in our ordinary speech. "Hearty", "heart-felt", "heartless", "cordial", all point to this in Saxon or in Latin.

Emotional states may either accelerate the rate or augment the force of the heart's action as in states of joy or excitement; or on the other hand they may depress and slow the heart and in extreme cases stop it altogether. This latter condition is called "total inhibition"; and great grief or great joy is equally potent. Old people have been known to succumb to emotional

[1] The worm-like movements of the muscle of the intestine are called peristalsis.

inhibition of the heart (syncope). Hence, we should be careful about telling these persons good or bad news very suddenly; suddenness is a factor in the grave issue. There was a day when it was dangerous to hand a telegram all of a sudden to susceptible people of this kind.

Blanching is an emotio-vascular reflex, it is an emotional stimulation of the vascular centre.

The *emotio-glandular* reflexes are equally familiar; they are typical of mentally induced tissue-activity. Weeping naturally occurs to one as an example of a glandular reflex preceded by emotion. Others are, emotional sweating, and emotional dry mouth, and inhibition of glandular activity.

The "cold sweat" of fear is an interesting reflex because it is unaccompanied by a vascular factor. Sweating usually occurs along with increased blood-supply to the sweat-glands, but in this reflex the glands are stimulated without the blood-vessels participating. This is possible on account of the separate innervation of these two systems.

Lastly, the emotio-metabolic is a large and rather ill-defined group.

Reflexes accompanied by emotion also

affect the state of the nutrition of various organs. Cases of the hair turning white through powerful emotion seem to be quite well authenticated; Darwin, in his *Expressions of the Emotions,* gives several instances. But according to Byron, the hair of the Prisoner of Chillon cannot be quoted as a case of this kind, for

> "It turned not white
> In a single night
> *As men's have turned* from sudden fears."

There is very little doubt that the hairs and nails can register emotional conditions. In persons who have come through a crisis, grooves or other markings on the nails may be detected, pointing to some antecedent interference with nutrition.

There are dentists who believe that, similarly, the teeth can bear evidence of a nutritional disturbance at some previous time.

These reflex emotional influences are of course not all of the depressant or morbid order; many emotional states exalt the nutritional state of the tissues and tend to stimulate their metabolism, as it is called. Such are referred to as "tonic" or "stimulating" conditions.

A happy frame of mind conduces to good

digestion and to a comfortable state of body; the pleasant emotion, in fact, has raised the tissue-tone and improved the assimilation.

Shakespeare has, of course, noticed this in the line—

> "Let good digestion wait on appetite,
> And health on both."

Finally, we come to the *ideo-motor* reflexes, to those bodily states which, certainly not volitional, are due to some purely mental state psychically higher than the emotion, and for which the term "idea" is sufficiently explicit. For our present purpose any state of mind not a sensation or an emotion or a volition is an "idea".

We know very well how ideas may take possession of the mind and express themselves in action apart from, and often in opposition to, the will. Such actions are ideo-motor reflexes. We distinguish in these the same four familiar groups—ideo-muscular, ideo-vascular, ideo-glandular, and ideo-metabolic.

Ideo-muscular reflexes are seen typically in the hypnotic state; the idea "suggested" is faithfully reproduced in the patient's mind and is there causal in inducing muscular activities or inhibitions.

If the hypnotized person is told to " march", he will march off at once, and on coming up against a blank wall will continue to march (" mark time ") until ordered to desist. Or the person hypnotized may be told to stretch out his arm, when it will become rigid, and rigid it remains for many hours, a state known as " catalepsy ". The whole body may be hypnotized into the condition of cataleptic rigidity.

The convulsions induced at the very idea of water, in the muscles of the jaw of a patient ill with hydrophobia, are ideo-muscular reflexes.

Ideas can also evoke reflexes in blood-vessels and glands as is seen in the hypnotic state. It is suggested to the sleeper that in due time he will awake cold; shortly he awakes with the blood-vessels of the skin constricted and he himself with all the marks of chilliness. Or he is told he will awake hot, and in due time he does so. Anyone who has witnessed these experiments would never maintain that the results are due to the patient's volition.

Lastly, when we come to the effect of ideas in metabolism we enter the vast field of mental healing. Possibly never before has this topic attracted so much attention as at the present time. Without accepting as beyond dispute the reality of all the "cures" announced at miracle-working spas, shrines or wells, or all the marvellous recoveries from illness described by the so-called "Christian Scientists", we must admit that there exists in the nervous system a mechanism whereby ideas can exert a potent and abiding influence on the bodily tissues and organs.

In 1911 I wrote in *Nerves*[1]—

"Psychotherapeutics is a department of the healing art likely to be more not less employed in the future." The use made of mental healing in the Great War proved how true was this prophecy.[2]

As there is a group of diseases called "functional" which are not due to any obvious or microscopic lesion but only to deranged innervation, so by restoring the healthy innervation, healthy function will be restored.

[1] Home University Library (Williams and Norgate).

[2] The subject of "Faith-Healing" or Mental Healing is more fully dealt with in my book, *Life and Science*, (Melrose), 1923.

HISTORY OF THE EVOLUTION OF THE CONCEPTION OF REFLEX ACTION

Previously to the emerging of the conception of reflex action, the notion of "sympathies" dominated the physiology of the nervous system.

When one part of the body seemed to act in consequence of stimulation to some other part, the two parts were said to be in "sympathy". It was at least recognized that the nerves were in some way involved.

René Descartes was the first to write of an involuntary action as "reflected". Descartes in his *Les passions de l'ame* (1646) pointed out that the cranial nerves were often involved in movements which were independent of the will.

His own words were—

"If one aims a blow at the eyes, even though we know he is a friend, and even if he does it as a joke and without doing us any harm, we at once, even against our will, close our eyes." It was the dissociation of this action, not from sensation but from volition, that arrested Descartes' attention.

His scheme of man as an automaton, set forth in great detail in his *De homine liber* is a celebrated attempt to emphasize what we now call reflex action ; but its physiology is almost worthless, as it was not based on experiments but evolved out of his own mind. He did a few experiments to verify it.

Descartes wrote in terms of "the soul" and "animal spirits" and "pores" in the brain and nerves.

The next step towards definiteness as regards reflex action was taken by the English physician and anatomist, Thomas Willis (1621-75), a pupil of our great Harvey.

Willis expressed himself thus (1659)—

"We may admit that the impression of an object driving the animal spirits inwards and modifying them in a certain peculiar manner gives rise to sensation ; and that the same animal spirits in that they rebound from within outwards in a reflected wave, as it were, call forth local movements."

From this simile, "as it were reflected", we have come to the conception of reflex action as we think of it to-day ; it is an example of the progress from the vague to the concrete in science.

The next step was made by Robert Boyle (1627-1691), the chemical philosopher. He reported that a decapitated viper, three days after the operation, still gave responses when its skin was pricked. His own words as regards its body are; "to be manifestly sensible of punctures being put into a fresh and vivid motion when it lay still before, upon being pricked".

The Rev. Stephen Hales (1677-1761), early in the eighteenth century, performed the fundamental experiment when he showed that after destruction of the spinal cord by pithing, no reflexes were elicitable.

The subject of reflex action was advanced by the Scotsman, Robert Whytt (1714-1766), of the Chair of Medicine at Edinburgh.

Whytt's discovery was that those "sympathies" did not need the integrity of the whole central nervous axis, but only a portion of it. He proved that the integrity of only one segment is necessary for any given reflex.

Whytt demonstrated that in order to elicit the reflex contraction of the pupil to light (Whytt's reflex), it is necessary only to have the anterior corpora quadrigemina intact.[1] Conversely, destruction of this region alone abolished the reflex.

Whytt discovered the phenomenon we now

[1] Two masses of grey matter included under Basal Ganglia.

call " spinal shock ", which is, that for some time after the frog has been brain-pithed or decapitated, no reflexes are elicitable from the cord. The reflex centres are inhibited by impulses descending on to them from the region so violently damaged. In about twenty minutes the shock wears off.

The discovery (1811-1822) of the separate functions of the two roots of the spinal nerves was an immense contribution to the conception of reflex action. For it made it quite clear that since all afferent impulses enter by the posterior roots, and all efferent ones leave by the anterior, these two roots must constitute integral parts of that reflex path which had not as yet received a special name.

The discovery of the respiratory centre by Legallois in 1826, and its confirmation ten years later by Flourens, served to render notions about reflex actions still more definite; for only in this bulbar centre have we a localized portion of grey matter through which reflexes, expressed as interferences with the rate and depth of breathing, can be brought about.

With the work of Marshall Hall (1790-1857) the conception of reflex action may be said to have been finally crystallized, for we find the term "reflex" used as though commonly accepted at the date (1833) of the publication of his Royal Society paper, "The reflex function of the medulla oblongata and medulla spinalis".

Dr Hall made a full study of the subject, and contributed many important additions to our knowledge. He gave us the terms "reflex nerve-arc", and "excito-motor", and showed that the maintenance of the state of closure (tone) of a sphincter muscle was reflex and due to the presence of a constant afferent factor.

Marshall Hall showed that all the following were essentially reflex actions—deglutition, vomiting, micturition and defæcation.

In 1837 Dr R. D. Grainger made a substantial contribution to the physiology of reflex action by insisting that the centres of spinal reflexion were in the grey matter of the cord and never in the white columns.

Before passing on to the "Conditioned Reflex", it would be well to become familiar with the conception of the Final Common Path as given to us by Sir Charles Sherrington.

In so far as this applies to a reflex action, it means that the reflex in question always employs the same efferent neuron and effector, no matter how many different afferent neurons and receptors have been used to produce reflexes through the centre. The case of the vomiting reflex (Fig. 10) will make this clear. V.C. is the vomiting centre in the Bulb, F. C. P. efferent neurons to the muscles of the stomach (*m, st*) and of the body wall (*m.b.w.*) respectively.

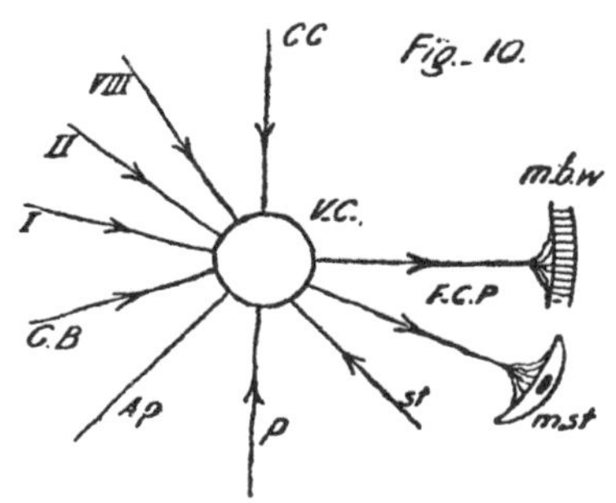

Scheme of the Final Common Path.

V. C. vomiting centre. F. C. P. efferent neurons from V. C. to muscle of stomach (*m, st*) and muscles of the body wall (*m. b. w.*). *St* afferent neuron from stomach. P from peritoneum, A*p*, from appendix, G. B. from gall-bladder.
I afferent neuron in nerve of smell, II in nerve of sight, VIII in nerve from semi-circular canals.
cc path from brain to convey impulses of emotional origin to V. C.

The commonest cause of vomiting is irritation of the mucous membrane of the stomach itself, but many other conditions of abnormality in such abdominal organs as peritoneum, appendix, and gall-bladder, for instance, may also induce it. Thus, the afferent neurons P, A*p*, and G. B. are called into activity. But further, vomiting may be caused by a smell or a sight or even by some emotional states when the nerve of smell or that of sight contains the afferent neurons.

Lastly, disturbances in the semi-circular canals involving neurons in the eighth cranial nerve are, as in sea-sickness, disagreeably effective in this reflex.

All these afferent neurons are involved in vomiting, but only the one set of efferent. The centre has many entrances, but only one exit.

CONDITIONED AND UNCONDITIONED REFLEXES

The Russian physiologist Pavlov and his pupils have carried out a very extensive series of experiments on reflex action whereby our knowledge of that subject has been widely extended.

Pavlov distinguishes two classes of reflexes, the " Unconditioned " or what one might call natural or non-acquired reflexes, and the " Conditioned " or acquired. The former group includes all the spinal, bulbar and cerebellar reflexes, those concerned with locomotion and the maintenance of the equilibrium, the knee-jerk, the eye reflexes, as well as those involving the blood-vessels, the digestive and the reproductive organs.

These are inborn ; they do not require to be learned, and they appear afresh, untaught, in each generation. They evidently include the " instincts ".

The character of the second group will best be learned from the description of an experiment. In a dog, the duct of the parotid gland (the salivary gland in the cheek), is brought to the surface of the cheek, and under antiseptic conditions is so fixed that the saliva flows not into the mouth but to the exterior of the body. When this wound has healed, the dog suffers no inconvenience whatever, and will stand up supported by straps in a specially constructed cage. If now the animal is given some food, there is at once the familiar reflex flow of parotid saliva which on the operated side drops from the duct into an apparatus which records the number of drops per unit of time. Now suppose that something is made to happen at the same time as the food is given, say a whistle is blown or a tuning-fork sounded, then, after a certain number of occasions in which the food and the musical note were presented together, the saliva will flow when no food is given but the whistle alone sounded. This reflex flow of saliva, which occurs after hearing, in this case, a musical note, is called " a conditioned reflex ".

All sorts of experiences may in this fashion be made to produce the reflex flow of saliva without any reference whatever to food. Thus, not only the smell of food, the sight of food, or the sight of the man coming with the food, but the rattle of a plate, a musical sound, and a flash of light, can all be made reflexly saliva-producing. This is what is called a " conditioned " reflex.

Equally interesting are the inhibitions. What is meant can be learned best from the following experiment. The conditioned reflex flow of saliva was being established by sounding a metronome while a dog was being fed. On one occasion, when the auditory stimulus was about to be given, the laboratory attendant began scraping away the snow from the steps of the building, with the result that the flow was at once stopped. The sound had distracted the animal's attention, and an inhibition was substituted for an excitation.

A vast number of occurrences in our every-day life are looked upon as conditioned reflexes. Further investigation into this subject would take us too far away from the A B C of nerves.

CHAPTER VI

THE TWO ROOTS OF THE NERVES

A mixed nerve is one in whose trunk are both efferent and afferent fibres, and the efferent fibres leave the spinal cord by the anterior root while the afferent enter it by the posterior. Each spinal nerve has these two roots; an anterior or ventral one and a posterior or dorsal with a distinct swelling on it. This swelling or "ganglion" consists of all the nerve-cells united to the fibres by T-shaped junctions.

The discovery that these two roots had different functions is the foundation of the physiology of the spinal cord; it is absolutely fundamental.

Taking the anterior root first (A R, Fig. 11), if this is stimulated by faradic electric shocks, convulsive movements of certain muscles will be produced. If the root is cut at 1, and the peripheral[1] end is stimulated, again muscular contractions take place; but when

[1] The portion on the lower or outer side of the cut.

the central end of the root is irritated, no observable results of any kind occur. From these results one would say that the root contained efferent fibres and that they were motor to muscles. This conclusion is confirmed by our finding that if the root is cut, the animal recovers from the operation with

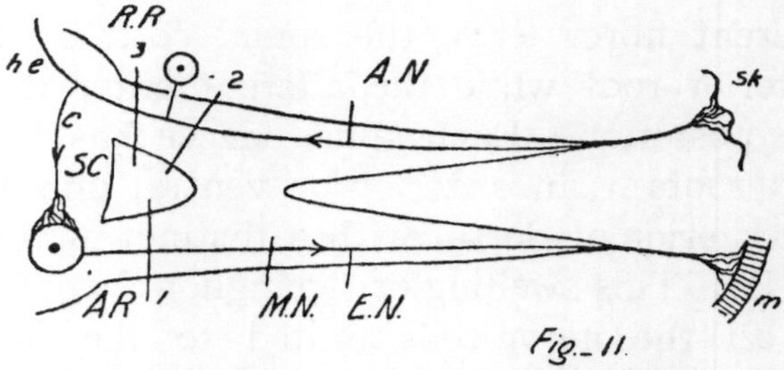

Diagram of the two roots of a mixed nerve (M.N.).

M, muscle; *sk*, skin; E. N. efferent neuron having left spinal cord (S C) by anterior Root, A R.
A. N. afferent neuron entering cord by Posterior Root P. R. *h. e.* headward extension of afferent neuron. *c*, collateral. 1, 2, and 3 sites of sections.

those muscles paralyzed which previously were convulsed when the root was stimulated.

Finally, the facts of Wallerian degeneration can be utilized, for if the anterior root is cut, and the animal allowed to live for a few days, then, on killing it and examining by means of the microscope the fibres in the mixed nerve (M.N.), a large number of fibres will be seen to be degenerated. These must have had their cells of origin in the spinal cord; and if regeneration is prevented, these cells will show Nissl's chromatolysis.

When the knife is going through the anterior root, no sensation or pain is produced, nor are there any reflex actions.

We may sum up and say:—

1. The anterior roots convey efferent fibres which are motor for muscles; and

2. The anterior roots convey no afferent fibres.

The posterior root shows us the opposite state of affairs. When one of the posterior roots is cut, at 2, Fig. 11, there is no paralysis of any muscle, but sensation in a certain area of skin becomes less acute, and if several adjacent roots are cut it is abolished. (Anæsthesia.)

Stimulation of the peripheral portion of the posterior root gives rise to nothing that can be observed[1]; whereas stimulation of the central end gives rise to reflex actions and evidently to pain as is shown by the animal's cries and distress.[2]

[1] The blood-vessel *b v* (in Fig. 8) may dilate (See page 94).

[2] The original experiments were done before chloroform was discovered, and they do not need to be repeated in any conscious animal.

Evidently the posterior root is conveying impulses inwards to the spinal cord.

The posterior root is for conveying impulses inwards not outwards, since nothing happens when it is cut and the peripheral end irritated.

Finally, if the root be cut between the ganglion (cell-bodies) and the cord at 3, Fig. 11, there is Wallerian degeneration into the cord as far up as the Medulla Oblongata, but not any in the fibres still attached to their trophic cells. As Wallerian degeneration is always in the direction of physiological conduction, this is an additional corroboration.

If the root is cut peripheral of the ganglion, at 2, Fig. 11, the peripheral portion degenerates, but the intraspinal part of the neuron does not.

We may sum up in this case and say—

1. The posterior root conveys impulses in an afferent direction.

2. The posterior root does not contain efferent fibres.

It was Bell's publications that first shed light on the double function of the nerve-roots. Bell was puzzled by the old view that the ganglia on the posterior roots blocked out sensory impulses, for every posterior root he had examined seemed to be for exactly the opposite purpose. It was something, he said, which could only be decided by experiment.[1] He did the necessary experiments on rabbits in 1810 and 1811 long before the discovery of chloroform, so that he could not prevent these animals feeling a little pain while he cut through the posterior roots. Later, he proved that so far from engendering pain, the cutting of posterior roots abolished sensation. No pain accompanies the cutting of an anterior root. He noticed that the animals with anterior roots cut were paralyzed in some muscles, and that there was no concomitant abolition of sensation ; and conversely, when the posterior roots were cut, there was abolition of sensation but no paralysis.

In 1822 the illustrious French physiologist, Magendie, repeated Bell's experiments and

[1] As it has been repeatedly said that Bell made his great discovery without experiments on living animals, and indeed merely by drawing conclusions from facts already known, it is necessary to quote his own words, which are to be found in a pamphlet entitled, *An Idea of a new Anatomy of the Brain*, printed in 1811. "An opinion prevailed that ganglions were intended to cut off sensation, and everyone of these nerves which I supposed to be the instruments of sensation have ganglions on their roots. Some very decided experiment was necessary to overturn the dogma." (Here follows a description of the experiment). "I now saw the meaning of the double connexion of the nerves with the spinal marrow."

greatly extended them, especially those on the posterior roots, so that the generalization regarding the two roots should be called " the Bell-Magendie Law ". It is the foundation of the modern physiology of the nervous system.

In its most modern phrasing the Law is—the fibres of the posterior root convey only ingoing or afferent impulses; any others are anti-dromic.

The fibres of the anterior root convey only outgoing or efferent impulses; any others are anti-dromic.

There is one phenomenon discovered long after the Bell-Magendic Law was established which at first sight seems as though it was an exception to that law. The main facts are somewhat as follow: if we stimulate the skin by placing some mustard, for instance, on it, the blood-vessels below that spot will be seen to flush. The familiar case is their flushing (dilating) after the application of a poultice. Now this looks like an ordinary vascular reflex action. That it cannot be a true reflex action is clear from the fact that the vessels can dilate after the posterior root is cut say at 2 or 3 in Fig. 11. A true reflex involves a centre—nerve-cells—in the central nervous system, but this is a purely peripheral affair.

The phenomenon is now known to be due to the fact that certain fibres divide at *d* into a branch X and a branch Y (Fig. 8). When, therefore, we stimulate an X branch, the impulses ascend to the division and descend the Y branch to the blood-vessel. This has been aptly called an "axon-reflex" or "*de*flex". The action of a poultice is thus explained.

CHAPTER VII

THE REFLEX MAINTENANCE OF TONUS AND POSTURE

A healthy muscle is firm to our grasp, it has what is called tonus; when unhealthy, it is soft and flabby, it has lost tone. In order that a muscle be maintained tonic, it must be constantly innervated from the central nervous system.

Destruction of the spinal cord at once abolishes the tone of the muscles of the limbs. A dead animal cannot stand on "all fours", it collapses; a corpse cannot stand on its feet.

This innervation of tonus is evidently an affair not requiring our conscious attention. The sphere of the maintenance of muscular tone is one largely outside that of consciousness. The tonus of muscles is not abolished by the removal of the cortex of the brain (decortication), indeed after this operation the muscles tend to become distinctly stiffer or "spastic", as it is called.

The fundamental mechanism for maintaining a muscle in proper tone is the integrity of its own muscle-to-muscle reflex arc; A^1 C B in Fig. 12. One proof of this is as follows: when one or two posterior roots of spinal nerves are cut, certain muscles are noticed to lose some of their tone. Now it is well known to physiologists that the cutting of sensory nerves from the *skin* does not result in a diminution of muscular tone, the reduction of the tone which follows on cutting the posterior roots must be due to the afferent fibres from the muscles themselves having been severed. The integrity of the muscle-to-muscle reflex arc has been destroyed, and the tone is at once impaired. The fundamental factor in the maintenance of tone is, then, a reflex one carried out by the proprioceptors of the muscle itself.

The grey matter of the brain has also some influence on the tone of muscles. As has just been indicated, in an animal from which the cortex has been removed on one side of the brain, the muscles of the opposite side of the body go into spasm and become abnormally rigid. This is explained by saying that in removing the grey matter of the brain, its unconscious inhibitory or restraining influence on the centres of the spinal cord has been done away with.

In disease of the brain, we have this state of matters illustrated. When in an apoplexy, the cells of the cortex have been destroyed or the fibres below them cut through or pressed upon, the same state of spasm of the muscles is produced. If now, instead of removing only the cortex, we remove the whole cerebrum (decerebration) and leave only the Bulb and spinal cord (bulbo-spinal animal), we shall then find that the extensor muscles in particular have gone into a state of spasm which gives to the animal a characteristically stiff attitude.

This condition, called "extensor spasm", is of such a nature that if a muscle be pulled out in the direction of bending the joint, it will remain in the new position instead of springing back into the original one. In the American phrase, "it stays put". Professor Sherrington, who discovered this decerebrate rigidity, has named the state of the muscle "plastic tonus". Once more a strongly inhibitory influence would seem to have been removed. According to most authorities, the source of this latter inhibitory influence is in one of these masses of grey matter towards the base of the brain, the Red Nucleus, one of the basal ganglia. At any rate, the cells responsible for the inhibition whose removal leads to plastic tonus are below the level of the cortex cerebri; so that it comes to this, that the proprioceptive spinal reflex on which muscular tonus fundamentally depends is influenced unconsciously both by cortical and by sub-cortical factors.

THE FUNCTIONS OF THE CEREBELLUM

The cerebellum, which is below the cerebrum and protected from its pressure by a stout sheet of connective tissue, is composed of two lateral portions, the hemispheres, and a single central mass (the vermis). Each half of the cerebellum is connected by many nerve-fibres to the cerebrum above, to the spinal cord behind, and to the brain-stem below, by the superior, inferior, and middle peduncles respectively.

The cerebellum sends nerve-fibres to the cerebrum by a crossed path (*s. c. p.*, Fig. 12), and the cerebrum sends fibres by a different and more roundabout crossed path (*m. c. p.*, Fig. 12) to the cerebellum. The reciprocal

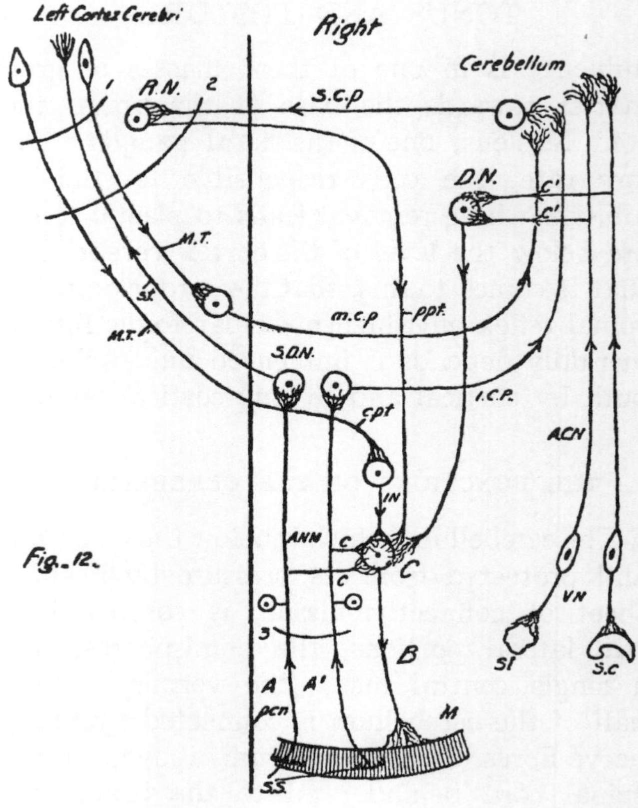

FIG. 12. Scheme of the cerebral, cerebellar and spinal factors maintaining muscular tonus.

A N M afferent neurons from muscle (*m*) taking origin in sensory spindles (SS) of muscle, one (A) leads to the afferent cerebral path via Sensory Dorsal. Nuclei of Medulla, S. D. N., the other A′ to the cerebellum via the Inferior Cerebellar Peduncle (I. C. P.)

A. C. N. afferent cerebellar neurons arising below the statolith (S*l*,) and in the semicircular canals (S. C.); en route to cerebellum these neurons give off collaterals (C′ C′) to Deiter's Nucleus D. N from which impulses descend to centres (in cord) C of the neurons (B) for the muscles. From the Red Nucleus (R. N.) impulses descend in the pre-pyramidal tract, (*p p t*) on to the same centre, C. The crossed pyramidal tract (*c. p. t.*) also sends impulses to the centre, C. The Cerebellum sends impulses to the Red Nucleus by Superior Cerebellar Peduncle (*s. c. p.*). 1, 2 and 3, levels of sections.

relations are of such a kind that when one half of the cerebrum, say the left, does not develop, the opposite or right half of the cerebellum remains undersized.

The cerebellum is abundantly related to the body through certain tracts of the spinal cord, the chief connection being with the skin and muscles of the body by tracts which do not cross (I.C.P., Fig. 12); that is, the left side of the body is represented in the left half of the cerebellum, and the right in the right. The right half of the cerebellum is therefore connected with the left half of the brain, but with the right half of the body. Now it will be remembered that the left half of the brain governs the right half of the body. The muscles of the head, neck and trunk are represented on both sides of the mid-line in the central parts of the cerebellum, those of the limbs in the lateral parts.

The cerebellum is late in appearing in the nervous system as we ascend the animal scale. As one might expect, it is relatively very large in the birds, creatures to whom the maintenance of an accurate balance is so very important. The fishes, for instance, have the cerebellum better developed than the reptiles, in which group it cannot have much functional importance.

Let us now try to make out what these various connections of the cerebellum with other parts of the nervous system mean. In the first place, injuries to or diseases of the cerebellum do not produce any impairment of a person's sensations. Animals from which the entire cerebellum has been removed, do not suffer any loss of sensation. A man with congenital, undeveloped cerebellum has no diminution of delicacy of sensation. The cerebellum is, therefore, not the physical basis of the elaboration of sensations, nor does it aid in that process.

But numerous nerve-impulses travel over the paths which reach the cerebellum through the spinal cord from the body (A^1 in Fig. 12) —impulses, therefore, which are afferent but not sensation-producing. The cerebellum *re*ceives but does not *per*ceive. Muscles, joints, skin, viscera, and those curiously complicated "semicircular" canals, a part of the internal ear, which have to do with balancing, all send their impulses to the cerebellum.

Figure 12 shows impulses from muscle to cerebellum by the route I. C. P. (Fig. 12), (inferior cerebellar peduncle), and from statocyst and semi-circular canals,[1] by afferent cerebellar neurons (A. C. N.). Impulses from joints, skin and viscera are not shown in this diagram.

The impulses from the semi-circular canals and the statocysts in the internal ear pass to the cerebellum of the same side by the afferent neurons of the vestibular nerve (part of VIII, Cranial of Anatomists) (V.N., Fig. 12). The details of the synapses on the path of these afferent cerebellar tracts (A.C.N.), which are very complicated, are not shown in Fig. 12.

Before these afferent tracts reach the cerebellum they give off collaterals which end over the cells of a nucleus known as Deiter's, whose neurons in their turn descend into

[1] In this elementary work no account has been attempted to be given of the special senses. One of these is that of orientation or the appreciation of our position in space, whether at rest or in motion. The statocyst with the statolith inside it is the end-organ related to our changes in posture, the semi-circular canals are similarly related on the afferent side to the movements of progression. The statolith is a minute concretion of limey material which presses on different spots of the lining membrane of the cyst according as the head is moved from one position to another. Some of the filaments of the afferent (vestibular) nerve take origin here. The semi-circular canals, filled with fluid, are curved tubes of membrane within bone, three on each side of the head, and so grouped in pairs that there is one pair in each of the three planes of space. Many filaments of the vestibular nerve arise in the lining of the canals.

the cord to end synaptically over the centres (C) for the muscles.

But the end-organs in skin, muscles, joints and the internal ear also send impulses which go to the cerebrum and give rise to sensations of different degrees of distinctness.[1] So that the state of affairs seems to be this: while certain organs send impulses to the brain to contribute to consciousness, these same organs simultaneously send impulses to the cerebellum, which do not give rise to consciousness. We cannot, therefore, speak of the cerebellum as being "aware" of anything; there is no simple word to express what exactly the cerebellum does as regards afferent impulses. It receives them from many parts of the body and "works them up" or correlates them without their arousing consciousness at all. The cerebellum receives afferent but not sensation-producing impulses, and, dealing with them subconsciously, relates them to outgoing impulses.

Let us in the next place see what is the state of affairs on the efferent or motor side. When a portion of the cerebellum is injured in an animal, the animal does not

[1] Those from muscle alone are shown on the neurons A and *st.* (this latter has had certain synapses omitted for sake of clearness).

suffer from paralysis of any muscles, but from a clumsiness of movement and an awkwardness of muscular action. The muscles have indeed rather less tone than before (atonia), and their movements are somewhat inco-ordinate or ataxic.

If the entire cerebellum has been removed, the animal cannot maintain its balance either in a state of rest or of motion; and if one half of the organ has been removed the animal has tremor of the muscles on that side, and tends to fall towards the side of the defect.

In man, injury to the cerebellum, according to its gravity, leads to more or less extensive inco-ordination of muscles, or ataxia, especially in the legs, so that the equilibrium of the body becomes unstable, whether the body is at rest or in motion. His muscles are not paralyzed, and he can move them voluntarily as before; but if the cerebellar disease is at all serious, he walks with a staggering gait like a drunken man, and strives to keep his legs far apart because this widens the base of support. This, of course, he does consciously; his straddling gait is the conscious compensation for the results of the subconscious irregularity in the cerebellar mechanism for the maintenance of the equilibrium of the body. The gait in cerebellar ataxia is characteristic, the head lags behind the torso, the torso behind the legs. Although, then, the cerebellum is not the seat of awareness of bodily states, and not the organ which originates bodily actions, yet it seems to be an important centre in the co-ordination of muscles which steady the body whether it is at rest or in motion.

The cerebellum sends no motor impulses to muscles or to any other " effector " organs, as far as is known. Efferent tracts do, however, leave it, not for the muscles directly, but for them indirectly, via the cerebrum. The path for this is by the superior cerebellar peduncle (*s.c.p.* Fig. 12), to the Red Nucleus, thence to cord centres by the prepyramidal tract (*p.p.t.*)

The cerebrum controls the muscles, decides whether they shall merely leave the body at rest or balance it as it moves about ; but all the time the cerebellum, in its turn, apparently controls or influences the cerebrum. For instance, it has been noticed that when the cerebellum has been injured, the cerebrum is apt to put forth either too little or too much nerve-energy, and so produce ataxia by deficiency or ataxia by excess (over-action, over-compensation).

The study of the behaviour of a large intelligent animal which has suffered the loss of one half of its cerebellum is instructive. Let us suppose that an adult dog has had its left cerebellar hemisphere removed; for the first few days it cannot stand properly but falls over on its left side. The eyes are not at rest but oscillating; the muscles of the left side are tremulous and rather weaker than usual, though by no means paralyzed. By degrees the dog gets better; its tremors are less severe, and finally it learns that it can prevent itself falling over if it walks towards the wall and leans up against it. This is the intelligent compensation for the defect of impaired maintenance of equilibrium; it is possible only because the animal's cerebrum is still uninjured.

Again, a dog with only half of the cerebellum intact, if thrown into the water, will swim more or less like a normal animal. It is noticed, however, that the dog does not go in a straight line, but in a curve which bends towards the sound side. The reason for this is interesting: dogs swim not like men, but by "grabbing" the water with their fore-paws. The muscles on the sound side, having more tone than those on the other, allow the paws to catch hold of the water better, with the result that if it is the left cerebellar half that is gone, the dog swims away towards his own right.

Muscles in human cerebellar disease are not paralysed, but they are tremulous, and to a greater or less extent show diminished tone and force. The same facts may be brought out by another device: if the dog above referred to is now made to walk on the hard ground, he is seen to be deviating towards his own left. This is because the right-sided muscles, having the better tone, get a better push-off from the ground than do the opposite ones, and so in time cause the animal to walk away from the straight line.

A curious thing was noticed about the dog made to swim. After a certain number of trials, it was learning to swim straight. The dog found that it could steer itself by means of its tail. It used its tail as a rudder curved in this case towards the left in order to bring its body over to the side from which it was drifting. A dog, whose *cerebral* hemispheres has been removed, cannot do this.

But the cerebellum receives impulses from

regions other than the periphery; it receives them also from the cerebrum. When the cerebrum is sending down nerve-energy to the muscles to maintain their tone or put them into activity, it sends simultaneously some energy over to the opposite half of the cerebellum (*m.c.p.*, Fig. 12).

The meaning of these various paths into and out of the cerebellum is probably somewhat as follows:

The cerebellum is informed of the state of tone or of contraction of the entire musculature of the body at any given instant; if, for any reason, it is necessary to increase that tone, the cerebrum has to emit fresh impulses, but just how intensely it must do so will depend on the amount of innervation which is sent over to it from the cerebellum (augmentor function). If, however, from any cause the cerebrum has been innervating the muscles too intensely, then it receives impulses from the cerebellum to restrain the intensity of its energy (inhibitory function).

The cerebellum is, as regards the cerebrum, a kind of "centrifugal governor": if the cerebrum is not doing enough in the way of innervating muscles, the cerebellum intensifies its activity; if it is doing too much, it cuts it down ; and all this below the level of consciousness.

The cerebellum is, then, not so much an organ for maintaining equilibrium as an organ corrective or regulative of the intensity of cerebral motorial innervation. This is what Hughlings Jackson meant when he taught that the cerebellum was for regulating continuous movements, while the cerebrum was for changing movements. The cerebellum is functionally an intermediary between the muscles and the cerebrum, but in order to be such, it must be constantly informed both of the state of the muscles and also of the cerebrum in regard to the output of energy from the latter. These conditions are fulfilled by the numerous afferent paths into it both from the muscles and from the brain.

A very great deal of our most recent knowledge regarding the physiology of the maintenance of the equilibrium is due to the researches of Professor Magnus of Utrecht and his co-workers. They have shown that the state of tension of a particular muscle-group determines reflexly the condition of those other groups whose co-ordinated activity underlies the maintenance of posture.

CHAPTER VIII

THE DOCTRINE OF CENTRES

The belief that there are "centres" in the central nervous system, that is, regions of grey matter devoted to particular activities, is absolutely fundamental. There is division of labour in the nervous system as in all other systems: one group of nerve-cells is for one form of activity, another for another. This division of labour means specialization of function. The centre for breathing is distinct from that for the heart's action, or for the tone of the blood-vessels, or for the secretion of gastric juice and so on. Nor can any one of these centres act vicariously for any other. If the centre for breathing could at any time become the centre for the heart's action or for the flow of saliva, there would be neural chaos.

The nervous system is the very reverse of a chaos, it is an exquisitely co-ordinated cosmos. The first differentiation in centres is into sensory or receiving, motor or emitting.

In this sense the cerebral centre for vision is a sensory centre; it is that receptive part of the cerebral cortex (occipital lobes) where seeing really occurs, for the eye, apart from the brain, does not "see". Some most unfortunate men in the Great War found this to be so when their occipital lobes were blown off. Their eyes, optic nerves and lower reflex optic centres were all intact, but because their sensory centre for vision had been destroyed they were blind, as blind as though they had no eyes at all.

There are centres for each of the special senses in that each sense is represented in a different cerebral region, the destruction of which abolishes the perceptions of that sense. Reception must precede emission; instruction go before performance; so that Shakespeare was absolutely right when he wrote—

> "Sense sure you have,
> Else you could not have motion."

The centre in the brain for touch is different from that for smell, for taste or for hearing, and so on.

But there are truly emissive centres, the best known of which are those for voluntary movements. The grey matter concerned in the emission of voluntary impulses is anatomically distinct from the sensory centres.

The sensory centres are the arrival platforms; the bridges and subways connecting these are the internuncial neurons in the commissures and other inter-central tracts.

If one portion of grey matter had to do duty both as sensory and motor centres, we should have the same confusion as when the one platform is used both for passengers arriving and for passengers leaving by the trains.

The anatomists use the term "centre" in a wider sense than do the physiologists. Every collection of nerve-cells (called a "ganglion"[1] by anatomists) is not a centre in the functional sense.

According to anatomists and histologists, any group of nerve-cells which gives rise to fibres is the centre for these fibres: such we call a "trophic" centre, because if the fibres are separated from the cells, the cells die.

The physiological definition of a centre is: a group of nerve-cells specialized to preside

[1] The term ganglion is now superfluous in the sense of a group of nerve-cells. In surgery it means a swelling on the sheath of a tendon.

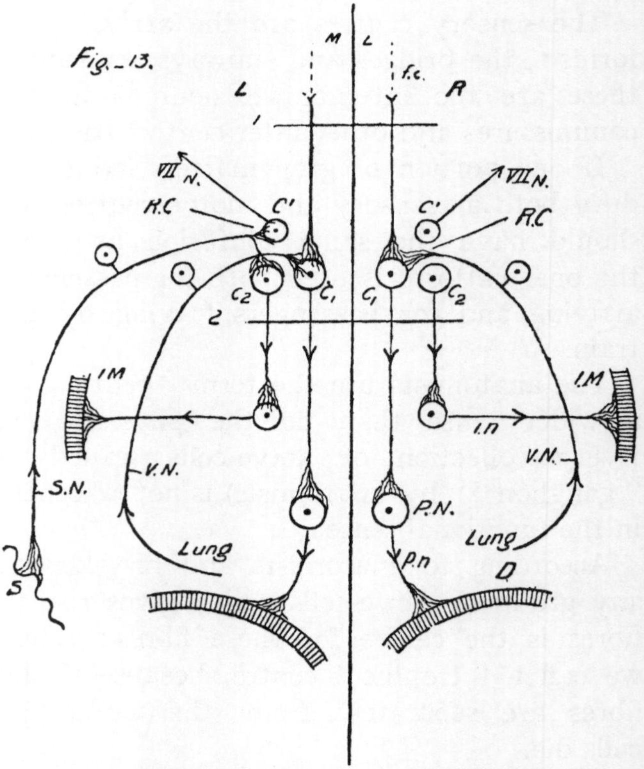

Diagram of respiratory centre (R. C.) in the Bulb. M. L. midline. C^1, cells sending impulses to muscles of nose, C_1 cells sending impulses to Phrenic Nuclei (P. N.) through *p. n.* (phrenic nerves) to diaphragm, D. (below the lung), C_2 cells discharging towards spinal cord centres for intercostal nerves (i. n.) supplying intercostal muscles (I. M).

V. N. afferent fibres of Vagus Nerve (X Cranial) arising in lung and ending in R. C.

S. N. sensory nerve from skin (S) sending impulses into R. C.

f.c. fibres from cerebrum descending on R.C.

over a particular function, that is to say, without whose presence that particular function cannot proceed.

Not all groups of nerve-cells are centres in this sense. Thus the nerve-cells (nuclei)[1] in the spinal cord which give rise to the phrenic nerves are not cells which preside over breathing, although they are the motor nerves to the diaphragm.

If the spinal cord be cut above the level of the cells trophic to the phrenic nerves at 2 in Fig. 13, the breathing ceases, although all that has been done is to isolate these phrenic nuclei from the influence of the Bulb. The phrenic nuclei (P.N.) and the phrenic nerves (*p. n.*) are still intact, but they are emitting no impulses to the diaphragm; therefore, they are not *the* respiratory centre. Anatomically the phrenic nuclei are a "centre", physiologically they are only a subsidiary, non-automatic, non-spontaneous centre.

An instructive example of a centre is the respiratory centre (Fig. 13) called by Flourens "*le noeud vital*" (the vital knot), because when it was destroyed breathing ceased at

[1] The "nucleus" of a nerve is an old term for the nerve-cells whose neuraxous constitute the axis-cylinders of the nerve in question.

once. It is a bilateral centre, for splitting the medulla oblongata in the mid-line does not compromise breathing at all (R. C. in Fig. 13). Destruction, however, on one side abolishes the movements of the diaphragm on that side.

Death by hanging is death by destruction of the respiratory centre by rupture of the medulla oblongata. When a man is " hanged by the neck till he be dead ", he is not suffocated by a rope tied round his neck, as many people imagine; he is suddenly suspended from his head by a rope fastened under the jaw, and the weight of the body ruptures the Bulb.

It will be profitable to examine a little more closely the physiology of the respiratory centre. The act of breathing is a double one; inspiration consists of raising the ribs and lowering the diaphragm, expiration of the opposite movements. Since no movements of these muscles go on in the absence of the intact Bulb, there must be in the Bulb a " centre for " initiating and maintaining the rhythmic movements of breathing. This respiratory centre appears to act automatically; and doubtless there is an element of independent activity within it, but we have proofs that it is under the influence of reflex stimulation.

In the first place, if the vagi nerves (V. N. in Fig. 13) be cut or frozen, the rhythm of breathing becomes very slow; at long intervals the animal takes a deep breath: this is followed by a long pause when there is no breathing (Apnœa).

Conversely, if we stimulate electrically the central end of the cut vagus nerve, we can hasten the abnormally slow rate until we restore the normal rhythm. Evidently there is a reflex nerve-arc, the afferent limb of which is in the vagus nerve, the efferent in the phrenic. The afferent fibres of the vagus or pneumogostric nerve arise partly in the lungs; so that it is the movements of the lungs themselves that are responsible for the afferent impulses which reach the centre by the vagus.

Afferent impulses from other internal organs can modify breathing, as for instance when there is peritonitis and in consequence pain from the descent of the diaphragm, the breathing is reflexly restrained.

But the centre can be stimulated reflexly in still other ways. We know how a dash of cold water on the skin—a plunge in the cold sea—makes one gasp, that is, take a sudden inspiration. Here the skin receptors have reflexly affected the inspiratory centre, stimulating it to a sudden, increased effort.

Occasionally a child is born alive (i.e. with beating heart), but it will not take its first breath. To get it to begin breathing it is smacked with a wet towel, so that the reflex we are alluding to is brought into play, and the respiratory rhythm thereafter maintained throughout life.

Sneezing and coughing are other respiratory reflexes. If the Bulb be cut across at the level 1, then a new rhythm known as the "Cheyne-Stokes breathing"[1] sets in. This consists of a rhythmic waxing and waning of the depth of the breathing until a period of no breathing is reached (Apnœa).

Thus, after the respiratory centre is separated from the cerebrum, it can still emit impulses so that the centre to some extent is independent of the regions of consciousness.

But of course it is very well known that the cerebrum can influence the respiratory centre as when we voluntarily interfere with our breathing, accelerate it, slow it or

[1] John Cheyne (1777-1836) and William Stokes (1804-1878).

stop it altogether. This is voluntary stimulation of the centre, and more or less voluntary inhibition of it, respectively. We can " hold " our breath if we will, but only for a very short time. Try as we may, we cannot prolong indefinitely this period of " voluntary apnœa ". After about a minute or so we experience a vague, disagreeable sensation of requiring air, of needing to breathe ; and we have to recommence breathing even against our will ; this is called " the breaking point ".

That emotions can influence the breathing is very familiar. One emotion can make the breaths " come fast " ; another can " take away the breath completely ".

So obvious is this that the ancient Greeks believed the soul to reside in the diaphragm, the word for which is " phren ". Hence, the terms " phrenology ", the curious pseudo-science of the mind ; frensy (properly " phrensy ") great agitation of mind, and " phrenopathia ", mental disease.

Sighing, laughing, moaning, groaning are all emotional modifications of the character or rhythm of respiration.

If all afferent impulses are cut off from the respiratory centre and the spinal cord be divided above the level of the cells of origin of the phrenic nerves, some impulses can still be observed coming from the isolated respiratory centre. For the movements of the small muscles at the nostrils continue to be made at the same rate as was that characteristic of the animal's breathing rhythm.

The respiratory centre is thus capable of acting spontaneously in complete anatomical isolation; it is, therefore, a real centre.

If an alleged centre is an independent centre, it should be capable of being stimulated in all of the following ways, namely by—

(1) Physical stimuli which include (*a*) mechanical, (*b*) electrical, and (*c*) thermal.

(2) Chemical stimuli.

(3) Neural stimuli which may descend from the cerebrum or be of a reflex nature. Both cerebral and reflex stimuli may be either tonic or depressant.

When mechanical stimulation in the form of increased pressure is applied experimentally to the Bulb, the breathing becomes slower. Nature performs this experiment for us when she creates what we call increased intracranial pressure as in tumours of the brain, compression of the brain, and certain other morbid conditions in all of which the respiratory rhythm becomes slower.

Another physical stimulus is heat, which in this case means blood reaching the centre at a temperature higher than normal. The demonstration of this is striking: the carotid arteries which supply the Bulb with most of its blood are placed within tubular, metal jackets, through which warm water can be circulated. As the temperature of the water rises and the blood gets hotter, the breathing becomes faster; the heat has stimulated the cells of the respiratory centre which respond by emitting their impulses at a faster and faster rate. The respirations are, however, shallower than normal. This sort of alteration in the breathing receives the name of dyspnœa, difficult or unpleasant breathing, in this case, heat-dyspnœa.

When we come to chemical stimulation, we come to the important subject of the chemical regulation of breathing. It has been proved experimentally that the tension of the carbon dioxide in the blood is the normal stimulus for inducing the depth of breathing, this gas being carried to the medulla oblongata in its arterial blood. Surprisingly small increases of the carbon dioxide in the blood are sufficient to bring about this result.

Chemical substances, other than carbon dioxide, for instance, lactic acid, can affect the respiratory centre. This acid, produced in excessive quantity in fatigue, produces rapid breathing or hyperpnœa. If the muscles of a dog be artificially fatigued by prolonged, powerful, electrical stimulation, and its blood injected into another dog, the latter will show signs of fatigue, one of which is rapid breathing.

Allied to the topic of stimulation of the respiratory centre by chemical agents, we have the peculiar affinity of this centre for salts of prussic acid. Hydrocyanic acid and its salts the cyanides are extremely deadly, in that they seize at once upon the living cells of the centre and immobilize them.

The rhythmicality of the respiratory centre is remarkable. The rhythm of discharge of volleys or salvoes of impulses at 18 to 20 in the minute in the healthy adult, is its chief characteristic. Day and night whether we wake or whether we sleep it holds on the even tenor of its phasic way during the whole term of our natural life. This rhythm is founded on the spontaneity of the activity of living matter modified by many conditions and agencies.

Our description of the respiratory centre may then be on this wise: it consists of two bilateral, symmetrically disposed groups of nerve-cells within the medulla oblongata, emitting at about 18 to 20 times a minute inspiratory impulses to the diaphragm and other muscles.

These cells are affectable by impulses—both conscious and unconscious—descending on to them from the cerebrum, as well as by impulses of a reflex character originating either within or at the surface of the body (for instance, skin S in Fig. 13).

The centre finally can be influenced by direct stimuli of a mechanical, thermal or chemical order. The centre possesses inherent rhythmicality modifiable by environmental conditions.

The accessibility of the respiratory centre to influences arising in various bodily states is evidently in the interests of the body as a whole; for it is imperative that carbon dioxide and water be eliminated from blood continuously; and that, occasionally, as the result of great muscular exertion, the excess of carbon dioxide should be got rid of as speedily as possible.

The respiratory centre is by no means the only one in the Bulb ; we may now enumerate some of the other centres there that have been recognized by physiologists :

The centre for the heart's action ; the centre for the blood-vessels ; the perspiratory centre ; the centres for the secretion of saliva, gastric juice and pancreatic juice ; the vomiting centre as well as centres for the bronchial muscle, the muscles of the stomach, intestine and gall-bladder.

These centres in the Bulb used to be called those of " vegetative life ", alluding to the fact that they innervated the vital organs outside the sphere of conscious governing.

Headward of the Bulb, there are in the mid-brain two important centres innervating muscles in the eye, the centre for the movements of the iris (pupil), and that for the muscle which focusses light on the retina.

CHAPTER IX

LOCALIZATION OF FUNCTION IN THE BRAIN

Our knowledge of localization of function in the brain was very late in coming. It dates from the years of the Franco-Prussian War (1870-71), when two army surgeons, Fritsch and Hitzig, used galvanic stimulation to the grey matter on the surface of the brain of a soldier whose skull-cap had been blown off. They noticed muscular movements on the side of the body opposite to the side of the brain so stimulated. Very shortly after their work was published, the late Sir David Ferrier, F.R.S., applied the faradic current to the exposed surface of the cerebral hemispheres of a large number of types of living animal. His researches, which have been abundantly confirmed, showed us that the cortex cerebri could be divided into three main regions of response, parts whose response was muscular movement, areas whose "response" was apparently some kind of sensation, and finally areas which gave no response at all, " silent areas", as they have been called.

For the first time in human experience it had been proved that the cortex cerebri was affectable, that is, accessible to artificial (electrical) stimulation. Haller, who died in 1770, Magendie (died 1855) and Fleurens (died 1867) all tried to simulate the living cortex cerebri by every kind of stimulation known to them—pressure, pricking, cutting, tearing, burning and by electricity—all without producing any effect. They therefore concluded that the living cortex was inexcitable, which agreed with Aristotle's declaration that the brain was " cold and bloodless ". In all probability these earlier investigators were operating on a brain already moribund, for unless loss of heat be avoided, and unless the full blood-supply be ensured, the cortical grey matter soon dies. It is also quite possible that what they stimulated was a sensory or even a silent area. Clinical observation *might* have told them that the cortex is responsive to such pressure as that of an intra-cranial tumour producing convulsions.

It would appear that the brain though

the "seat" of consciousness is not sensitive to mechanical damage to itself. Ferrier records the specific case of the excision of the centre for vision in a monkey without eliciting any pain.[1]

The passage is: "the angular gyri were seared with the cautery without further narcotization and without the slightest sign of pain or discomfort on the part of the animal".

Headache is due to tension or inflammation (meningitis) in the membranes of the brain which are supplied with nerves of pain but not of ordinary sensation.

Ferrier's work gave the first experimental proof in the case of a lower animal that the cortex did not act as a whole, but that there were differentiated in it both motor regions and sensory regions.

Stimulation of the motor regions of the cortex evokes co-ordinated movements of limbs, not merely contractions of isolated muscles.

The sensory areas were naturally much more difficult to discover, for in the nature of the case one had to interpret the subjective sensations of an animal. Ferrier

[1] Ferrier, *The Functions of the Brain*, 2nd edition, 1886, p. 278.

had to infer, for instance, that he was stimulating the centre for vision when the animal turned its head and eyes in a particular direction as though seeing something, and the centre for hearing when it pricked up its ears, as though trying to hear something, and the centre for smell when it dilated its nostrils as though smelling something. There is much evidence from Pathology and Medicine that corroborates the existence both of motor and sensory centres.

Thus, a cerebral tumour, a depressed bone or a foreign body under the skull pressing on some one of the motor areas will give rise to twitchings of such muscles as are innervated by the area pressed upon. By noting carefully in which muscles the twitching begins, the surgeon has been able to cut down on a tumour pressing on the centre for these muscles, and on excising it to relieve the symptoms. The surgeons use a map representing on the outside of the skull the various motor centres in the cortex below.

Fritsch and Hitzig noticed that if they applied the electrodes to certain spots for too long a time, there was a spread of the activity from the muscles in which the twitching had begun to more distant groups. This indicated a spread of the cellular excitement from the spot stimulated to adjacent areas. This is alluded to as Artificial or Stimulation Epilepsy.

There exists a clinical condition which is its counterpart.

In certain cases of brain disease, careful observation shows that a twitching may begin in a single muscle, for instance, of the thumb or forefinger, and thereafter spread until the fingers, wrists, forearm and arm are all sharing in the convulsions.

This condition is called "Jacksonian Epilepsy" after the distinguished neurologist, Dr Hughlings Jackson (b. 1834, d. 1911), who first described it in 1875. By noting the muscle in which the convulsion begins, the surgeon can frequently cut down on the centre for that muscle and, finding a tumour there, excise it. This was done repeatedly by Sir William MacEwen and Sir Victor Horsley within a few years of Ferrier's work being published.

Though of course muscles are paralyzed when their cortical centres are destroyed, yet the localization is of *movements* as such rather than of isolated muscles. The muscles are paralyzed in that they cannot be made to move by any volitional effort. The will is there, the desire to move muscles is as strong as ever, but because the physical basis of the will is absent, the muscles cannot be moved. The will cannot " act " on nerve-fibres severed from the cortex. The cortex cerebri is the organ of the will.

The excision of the area for a muscle or group of muscles is in reality " the control experiment " to the excitation of that area. The muscles paralyzed by severance from their cortical centres do not waste away as do muscles whose trophic centres in the spinal cord are destroyed. The former grey matter has, therefore, been called " the highest trophic realm ", and the latter the " lower trophic realm ".

The cortical motor centres are so related to the segments of the body that the centres for the toes and feet are highest, and those for the face lowermost in position.

It was found that this cortical representation of muscular movements was far more detailed in the case of muscles involved in fine or precise movements than in those whose performances are simpler and more massive. Thus, the area for the face and hand muscles is much larger than that for the whole of the muscles of the back. The cortical representation is on a functional, not an anatomical, basis ; so that the physiological endowment of the small muscles of the face and hands is vastly richer than that of the large muscles of the back which merely maintain the upright posture. The more numerous and delicate the performances of which muscles are capable, the larger and more detailed will their cortical representation be.

Ferrier next established a very important point in that the same localizing effects could be got by stimulating the white tracts below the grey matter ; and that the precise movements elicited differed in this latter case according as the electrodes were moved about from point to point just as happens when the grey matter itself is stimulated.

This very important experimental observation is of course the proof that the white fibres under the cortex are the conducting strands for nerve-impulses which have originated above.

The way to complete the demonstration that an area of cortex is the centre "for" a muscle is to excise that area and find that we have produced paralysis of the same muscle which was thrown into activity by the stimulation of that area. This was done by Ferrier, Schäfer, Horsley, Beevor and others.

It would be a mistake to suppose that only contractions of the muscular groups arise from cortical stimulation, for quite often it is inhibition or a quelling of tone (muscular relaxation) which takes place. Sir Charles Sherrington in particular has demonstrated this phenomenon: there is, in other words, cortical representation of muscular relaxation (inhibition) just as there is of muscular contraction.

The movements which are elicited by artificial stimulation of the motor areas are very evidently those which are carried out by volitional effort in the intact animal. They correspond to those which in the human being are acquired, learned, specialized, co-ordinated; and it is these which are the first to disappear in destroying lesions of the cortex cerebri and of the efferent system.

The functional indispensability of the cortex is revealed when we consider the time element in stimulation of the cortex and of the white matter below it.

If the cortical area for the fore-paw of a dog is stimulated, and the time elapsing between the moment of stimulation and that of contraction is marked on a suitably fast moving surface, the time-interval is found to be 0.065 of a second. But if, now, the appropriate point below this in the white matter is stimulated, the time interval is shorter, 0.045 of a second; the difference (0.04 of a second) is much too long to be taken up by the travelling of the impulse through the very short distance from the surface to the point below where the white fibres were stimulated. This period of time—the time of cortical delay—must be due to the functional presence of cells of the grey matter. It is comparable with the "time of spinal delay" in a reflex action.

It has also been shown that in a dog drugged with morphia or other narcotics, the time of cortical delay is much longer than in the undrugged state which is a subtle way of showing that the brain cells are causal in the emission of impulses.

The demonstration that centres for sensation exist in the cortex cerebri was another very important discovery by Ferrier.

His method was first of all to stimulate an area and obtain such results as led him to believe that it was the seat of a particular variety of sensation ; and then, as a control, to excise that area and find that the sensation in question was abolished. Macacque monkeys were used because, owing to their relatively high intelligence, they were clearly more suitable than animals less mentally endowed, but the results were confirmed, in so far as that was possible, on dogs, cats and jackals.

Let us take first the case of sight ; the region concerned is that known to anatomists as the occipito-angular. When this region was stimulated (on one side) the animal turned its eyes, and sometimes its head also, to one side as though it were observing something in the field of vision, and the pupils were noticed to have contracted. These things must be interpreted as meaning that the electrical stimulation of this zone gave rise to what is called in human psychology a hallucination or a subjective vision of something in consequence of which the animal, imagining it saw this thing, turned its head and eyes to get a better view of it. All these movements, including the contraction of the pupil, are such as would be made by an animal looking at something that had engaged its attention.

The converse effects after removal of the centres were equally instructive. When only one occipito-angular region was destroyed, the blindness was only partial; both regions had to be removed before the blindness was total and permanent. Ferrier's description of the utter helplessness of the monkey is very striking: after double removal it had to depend entirely on smell and touch for information about its food, neither of these senses being in any way impaired.

The discovery of the centres for hearing was made on exactly similar lines. The stimulation of a region on the side of the brain caused the monkey to turn its head, prick up its ears and even open its eyes as though it heard something. Its attitude was exactly that which Ferrier had previously noted in the intact monkey as the result of a loud noise.

To produce total deafness, the whole of certain convolutions on both sides of the head had to be excised; and when this was done the animal was quite unable to hear the loudest sounds, no matter how close to the ear.

By similar experimentation, the cerebral seats of most of the other senses have been explored; and we are not at all surprised to know that the centres for the senses of smell and taste, so closely associated in our experience, are situated very close to each other in the brain.

While the anatomical and physiological independence of the sensory centres has thus been established, it is perfectly clear that when in action those sensory centres must be in the most intimate and immediate relationship. On the anatomical side this requires a great profusion of connecting (commissural or inter-nuncial) fibres, and immense numbers of such are known to exist. Even when a single object is viewed and recognized, the psychologists tell us that a large number of qualities are simultaneously perceived, which on the physiological side means that a number of sensory centres are simultaneously in action. The fullest possible provision is made for this linking up of the several senses, so that the old saying "the brain works as a whole" is quite true.

Lastly, as regards localization, there are areas from which no response can be obtained upon electrical stimulation—the "silent areas". Physiological psychologists believe that these regions are the anatomical bases of all those characteristically human mental processes we group under the term "thinking". In the human brain, when we have assigned the areas for movement and for the various sensations, we find relatively very large areas corresponding to the silent areas of the monkey and still lower animals. In the human brain these are called "association centres".

Tumours and other pathological conditions are what we must depend on in the case of man for information regarding all problems of cerebral localization; and in so far as the results of electrical stimulation of animal brains can throw light on human conditions they are entirely corroborated by clinical observations.

If we compare the brain of man with that even of the highest ape, we shall be struck with the relatively large amount of association areas present in the former, which agrees, perfectly, of course, with his intellectual pre-eminence.

These non-motor, non-sensory areas are called "associational" since they are without doubt the cerebral bases of all the higher forms of thought of which the data or raw materials are sensations, and which inevitably sooner or later overflow into action. The German neurologist, Flechsig, has studied the dates at which the neurons of these "silent" areas acquire their medullary sheaths; and he found that this always occurs much later by many months than it does in the motor and sensory areas. The pre-eminently human function of speech we shall shortly see is one which involves associational centres; these are, therefore, really the physiological basis of educability.

The largest of the association areas is that known as the pre-frontal, the portion of the cerebrum behind the forehead and overlapping the eyeballs. Here, if anywhere, intellect, the reason, the "mind" have their seat. It is this region which is so poorly developed in congenital idiots, so well developed in men of great mental capacity.

Mere size, however, does not necessarily indicate intellectuality, it is the number and depth of the sulci (depressions) that do so.

It has, indeed, been found that when the frontal lobes are well developed, the sulci in all parts of the brain are numerous and deep. In the female brain the frontal lobes are smaller than in the male, and the sulci are not so well marked. A few female brains have well marked sulci like the male; and, contrariwise, some male brains in this respect have female characters.

The cerebral localization of emotion as distinct from sensation, volition, or the purely intellectual activities, has remained an unsolved problem. If "emotion" as a term is objectionable, the expression "affective state" may be substituted.

It was at one time believed because such affective states as pleasure, satisfaction, pain and such vague sensations coloured with "affective tone" as desire for food, water, air and "sex" had no discoverable cortical locus, that they had no cerebral basis at all.

This view is probably a mistaken one. The large basal ganglion called the Optic Thalamus is now believed to be that (subcortical) part of the cerebrum related at least to painful emotions. There seems to be no corresponding locus for pleasurable states (Euphoria).

As there are receptors for pain, specific and separate nerves for pain, in the spinal cord, and paths conducting pain-producing impulses it would seem quite in agreement with these things that there should be a central region set apart to receive the impulses which have travelled over this pain-related system.

The Optic Thalamus is now regarded as the head ganglion of painful states.

It has been asserted that in certain cases of excessive, persistent and incurable pain, the Optic Thalamus has been found post mortem to have been the seat of gross lesion.

CHAPTER X

THE FUNCTIONS OF THE CEREBRUM SPEECH: PHRENOLOGY

We have seen that the cortex cerebri is "the organ of the mind", as Bastian put it years ago. The cortex nowadays, however, is often referred to as the neo-pallium, a term which refers to its late appearance in the animal series.[1]

If we arrange the animal series thus, fishes, reptiles, amphibia, birds and mammals—we may observe that the pallium or mantle over the basal ganglia occurs only in the last three groups. In the fishes and reptiles there is no pallium over the basal ganglia, of which the optic thalamus is the most prominent. In these animals the optic thalamus is the end-station for the sense of vision, so that such consciousness as is aroused by the optic stimuli must be related to the grey matter of this ganglion. In the

[1] The words mean "new cover": neo, Greek, for new, pallium, Latin, for a mantle.

case of the fishes, sight and the power of balancing are of course the two most important functions which lead to locomotion and the acquiring of food. But it is very clear that what we mean by mind—educability, the power of originating new forms of activity, and of memory—is not to be found in animals so lowly as fishes and reptiles; to speak of the mentality of a fish is absurd.[1]

In the amphibia, e.g. in the frog, the neopallium is very small and smooth; but, small as it is, it is the basis of such power of origination as the animal possesses. A frog from which the cerebral hemispheres (neopallium) have been removed (decerebrate frog) will live for months, but it sees nothing and hears nothing; it will starve rather than feed itself. Objects have no "meaning" for it; it will swallow food placed in its mouth, but it would sit where it is forever.

It is not paralysed: when thrown into water it swims, and it has retained all its reflexes; but surrounded by food it would starve; and it never makes any attempt to escape from its place of confinement. It is in a state of complete mindlessness.

[1] The amount of memory in the fish is very small; a fish just pricked by the hook of the angler, will return again and again until finally caught.

Similar is the behaviour of the bird, the pigeon, for instance, which has had its cortex cerebri removed. This (decorticated) bird can be kept alive indefinitely with appropriate care and feeding, for the bird itself will not feed itself spontaneously. It can walk and fly and perch on a narrow support; but it cannot escape from danger. When placed on a hot plate, it raises one leg, then the other, and finally squats down where it is; it never flies away. It sits all day in a dozing attitude with eyelids closed and head drawn in. It would be best described as a very stupid, lethargic bird, which originates nothing, does nothing to avert danger, and cannot feed itself. The neo-pallium in the bird is evidently the basis of those reactions to the environment which underlie the so-called "instinct" of self-preservation and the search for nourishment. The sex-instincts are annulled, for though the decorticated male pigeon will "coo" incessantly, he will take no notice of the hen bird when placed close beside her. All spontaneity is gone.

Coming now to the mammal, it is found that a dog, for instance, cannot survive the operation of decortication done all at one time. Portions of the cortex, therefore, have to be removed at long intervals. This, the method of Goltz, is to wash away the grey matter piecemeal by a powerful stream of water. Such a decorticated dog lived for one and a half years. Once more we see the same absence of spontaneity; food placed near it is unrecognized; only when very hungry and when its nose is actually in contact with the food will it eat any of it. The animal at first is, of course, paralyzed, but it recovers its powers of walking and is in fact very restless. The conspicuous thing about Goltz's dog was "its lack of intelligent response": painful stimulation to the skin evoked growling, but no biting; threatening measures called forth no fear, no anger; caressing it evoked no pleasure. The animal had no intelligence, no spontaneity, and had lost interest in life. Observation of this decorticated dog leaves us in no doubt that the neo-pallium is the organ of the mind.

Surveying the animal series we come to the same conclusion, no neo-pallium, no mentality; and the more neo-pallium, the more mentality.

This mantle of grey matter is *new*, because in the evolutionary history of animal forms it was late in being super-added to the basal ganglia, the seats of reflex responses to environmental stimuli. It grew upwards, forwards and backwards, covering the older structures beneath.

One of the cerebral structures old in the history of vertebrates is the olfactory lobe—the central organ of smell. Fishes have large olfactory lobes. Animals which have the keenest sense of smell have this olfactory lobe the most largely developed.

The cells composing the neo-pallium are not by any means all of the same type; histologists have come to describe three main layers in it, known, respectively, from above downwards as the supra-granular, the granular, and the infra-granular layers.

The name "granular" is an old one and referred to the appearance of myriads of small cells which looked like granules or dots in the field of the microscope. These cells are known to be receptive (sensory) and distributing in their nature. In fact, they distribute impulses towards the supra-granular layer, and they themselves receive an immense number of different fibres.

The infra-granular layer is of remarkable constancy of form in all types of mammalian brain. Never absent from any human brain, it is as well marked in the feeble-minded as in the most intellectual person. It is the first cortical cell layer to be laid down and the first to attain to structural maturity. Neurologists and psychiatrists have no doubt that it is the layer subserving the animal instincts, those of self-preservation and of sex, the search for food, drink and shelter. It is the neural basis of the innate, of those actions or dispositions which require no education, training, teaching or previous experience. Professor R. J. A. Berry, M.D., who has studied the brain in great detail, speaks of this layer as the region of the "instinctive reflexes of men and the lower animals".

Very sharply contrasted with all this is the supra-granular layer. It is the layer which distinguishes the human from the infra-human type of cortex; it is the anatomical basis of the superiority of man.

In all forms of feeble-mindedness it is poorly developed; and it is degenerated in those forms of mental derangement we group under dementia. It is the physical basis of educability, of mentality and of mental acquisitions. It is the region which underlies experience.

At birth it is only one half of the thickness which it will ultimately attain ; its neurons will continue to increase in size and complexity, to have their collaterals, processes, arborescences, and synapses become more and more intricate as time goes on. This layer and these processes are the cellular ground-work of the Association of Ideas.

The supra-granular layer in infra-human brains is very much simpler in its details. It is the layer of memory, of the revivability of those " traces ", motor and sensory, which have been laid down within it.

Function is, then, truly localized in the cerebrum, in that not only do different areas subserve different mental activities, but different strata do this also : function is stratified in the neo-pallium.

The motor areas are recognizably different from the sensory : this was the particular contribution to the subject of localization made by Dr A. W. Campbell in his magnificent work on microscopical appearance as a guide to localization of function (1905). Campbell was able to show that the minute structure of motor centres, sensory centres and association areas was different in each and characteristic of each.

Coincident with this cellular growth in complexity is the growth in surface-area which is so marked by the infolding of the cortex—the formation of sulci, as the anatomists call them.

Up to the twentieth week of intra-uterine life, the human hemispheres are smooth, closely resembling the state which is permanent in the guinea-pig. The area of the human cortex at forty years of age is many times larger than what it was at birth.

In the adult male, the average area of the neo-pallium is 2,352 square millimetres or 1.5 square feet. The cortex cerebri in man is from 2.5 to 3.5 mm. thick, and this has been estimated to contain 9,250 million cells. The weight of the entire cerebrum is from 1,360 to 1,488 grammes or 1.5 kilogrammes ($3\frac{1}{3}$lbs.): in idiots it is frequently less than 2 lbs.

SPEECH

The power of speech distinguishes mankind from all lower types however " anthropoid ". As an articulatory performance, the " talking " of the parrot is remarkable, but we are perfectly sure that there is no cerebration underlying it comparable with the human expression of ideas we call " speech ". We cannot investigate the cerebral aspect of speech without first looking a little into some of the sensory centres in the cortex. The centres for any one sense are not all exactly on the same functional level; there are lower sensory centres and higher sensory centres.

Let us take first of all the sense of vision. By the lower sensory centres we mean that part of the occipital lobe which is the physical substratum of our seeing light, that is of our consciousness of liminosity, form and colour, a kind of centre possessed by all animals which have eyes and a cortex cerebri. In this there is nothing characteristically human.

But there is a much higher visual centre, one having to do with the appreciation of the *meaning* of what is seen; a portion of the cortex which evidently requires to be *educated* before it can perform its functions. It is the centre for the recognition of objects, persons, scenes; in fact it is the visual memory centre. A portion of it is the centre we educate when we learn to read.

This higher visual centre is one of the " silent areas " which have been called "association centres". Such a functional name is appropriate. Since the higher visual centre is so pre-eminently occupied with the sight of words and their meanings, it is called the Visual Word Centre. Dr Campbell has shown that the microscopic structure of the lower visual centre is recognizably different from the higher.

An exactly similar state of matters holds good with reference to the cortical centres for hearing. Here there is an auditory centre which all animals with a cortex possess, and also a higher one peculiar to man, the Auditory Word Centre. Again, it has been shown that there are microscopic differences between them. In point of fact, the heard word-centre is one of the first centres educated or at least employed; for it is a question if we may call "educated" a person who has learnt by ear only his mother-tongue. The most illiterate and the feeble-minded will use this centre to speak their native language, which they can neither read nor write. Normally, of course, the heard word-centre is utilized to register intelligent heard word-memories—the meanings of words—and it is used along with the seen word-centre as soon as the child learns to read. The seen word-centre and the heard word-centre are, as might be supposed, closely connected together by many commissural fibres. Together they act as one of the most important association-centres of the human brain—the physical basis of the appreciation of the sensory data for speech.

It is quite evident that in learning to speak, the child merely imitates certain sounds it hears from time to time. The mother, the nurse, and the brothers and sisters, convey to the growing brain those impulses which in the heard word-centre acquire in due time more and more meaning and become heard word memories. It is a very familiar fact that if the child is deaf, it will later be dumb, for if it cannot hear words, it cannot imitate them, and its ideas must be expressed in some other way than by the muscles of articulation, by those of gesture or " pantomime ", as it is called.

The normal route for speech as a sensori-motor mechanism is ear, lower hearing centre, heard word-centre, motor speech centre, and finally the bulbar centres for innervating the muscles of articulation in the lips, tongue, cheeks and palate. If this route cannot be begun to be traversed owing to deafness, then the child must be a "deaf-mute"; it is deaf and dumb, dumb because deaf.

The usual course of events in education is that the child will be "taught his letters", that is, taught to read by a process involving the seen word-centre and the motor speech-centre. He early associates the sight of the letter B, for instance, with the sound "bee" as pronounced by his teacher and himself, so that this "learning to read" is, for the young child, a process of the most arbitrary association of sights with sounds which he himself has been taught to produce.

It is therefore clear that there must be a portion of the brain which is functionally a motor speech-centre—an association-centre—not the cortical motor centres for the muscles involved in articulation but a functionally higher centre which, being instructed by the heard and the seen word-centres, discharges impulses down towards the motor centres.

Speech as a motorial cerebral activity requires a motor centre, a centre to receive the sensorial and to discharge the motorial. The motor speech-centre is such an executive centre.

It is interesting to know that the existence of such a speech-centre was, in point of time, the first centre to be inferred in the human cortex, and that long before Ferrier's day, and long before the conception of cerebral localization of function had arisen.

It was J. F. Gall, a German physician, who, after much study of the subject, came to the conclusion that speech must be a function of the brain and of a more or less localized region of it. His general argument was somewhat as follows: the main difference between man and the lower animals is the relative amount of brain (cortex) in each respectively; intellect, therefore, has its physical seat in the cortex, and speech is *the* mental capability which distinguishes man from the lower animals.

Gall went further than that, for he definitely localized the speech centre, a centre for the memory of words—" in that region resting on the posterior half of the roof of the orbit between the anterior border of the third Frontal convolution and the posterior border thereof abutting on the fissure of Sylvius, is the organ of the memory of words".

These are Gall's own words, and they show how definite were his views on this subject.

The discovery of the speech-centre is nearly always attributed to the French anthropologist, Paul Broca ; but there is no doubt that nearly forty years before, Gall had come to the conclusion that some one part of the human cortex cerebri was the material substratum of speech in the same sense that some other part of it was the region in which intelligent guidance of certain corresponding co-ordinated muscular activities was located. Gall was enormously handicapped by not possessing the corroborative knowledge that the cortex is a living tissue exactly as is a muscle or a gland, and in virtue of its vitality is performing functions as definite as they. He studied cases where injury to the brain resulted in abolition of the power of speech or " aphasia ", as it is called ; and was fully convinced that speech was a function of the cerebrum, and therefore must have a locus. He located it in the frontal lobes over the eye-balls, and believed that men who were great linguists had exceptionally large development of the frontal lobes, which made itself obvious in the conformation of the face. As is well known, he was thence led into what was later named " Phrenology ", a pseudo-science, yet one containing more than the proverbial grain of truth amid the error.

Had the physiology of Gall's day been equal to assimilating his teaching as regards the cerebral localization of the power of speech, cerebral physiology itself would have been much earlier illuminated, and Gall might not have been led by the will-o'-the-wisp of "cranioscopy", into the morass of bad physiology where he was dragged by his energetic, but ill-informed lieutenant, Spurtzheim.

The Frenchman J. B. Brouillard in 1825 connected speechlessness with disease in the anterior lobes of the brain; and in 1836 Marc Dax first reported on the frequency of speechlessness with right-sided paralysis.

Paul Broca (b. 1824, d. 1880), the physician and anthropologist, in 1861 published his first case describing aphasia as the result of disease of the brain, but unaccompanied by the paralysis of any body-muscles.

The motor speech-centre is evidently, paradoxical as it sounds, one of the "silent areas", if we assign to it a level in the functional hierarchy. It commands the motor areas for the movements of the muscles of articulation; and it itself receives impulses from the heard word-centre and the seen word-centre.

In cortical or " Pure " Aphasia, there has usually been some interference with the blood supply to the Frontal lobe causing a localized anaemia. The motor speech-centre is therefore functionally incapacitated, and the power of expressing ideas in words abolished. There is no paralysis of the muscles of articulation (anarthria), and none of any body-muscles. It is a purely cerebral defect ; the centre responsible for the emission of impulses to the motor areas for the duly co-ordinated movements of muscles is out of action. Often the cause of the cerebral anæmia is a small clot of blood blocking up a branch of the middle cerebral artery ; but there are some cases where the cause of the anæmia is more obscure probably because toxic.

In this " pure aphasia " the power of writing is retained so that the patient can express his idea through that medium. This was evidently the form of aphasia which afflicted Zaccharias the father of " John the Baptist " (Luke i. v. 63), for it is recorded that on being asked the name which the child was to have, he *wrote,* " His name is John ". When this faculty is lost, the patient must have recourse to gesticulation, and signs, or pantomimia.

Instead of the abolition of intelligible speech the use of the words may be retained, but they are strung together in a meaningless order called "jargon speech" or paraphasia. This is evidently what Shakespeare is describing in *A Midsummer Night's Dream* in the lines—

> "His speech was like a tangled chain,
> Nothing impaired, but all disordered."

The other variety of speechlessness is subcortical aphasia, the kind produced by a lesion—usually a blood-clot—pressing simultaneously upon fibres for the muscles of articulation and for those of the limbs. The level where these adjacent fibres are thus pressed upon is known to anatomists as the "Internal Capsule". Owing to the opposite-sided relationships of cerebrum and muscles, a lesion in the left Internal Capsule produces along with the aphasia paralysis of the limbs on the right side of the body.

The muscles are paralyzed in the sense that they cannot be reached by the volitional impulses; but their tone is not abolished because the trophic centres of their nerves are still intact in the Bulb and spinal cord respectively. Thus in subcortical aphasia there is not that disfiguring one-sided paralysis of the cheek and lips such as occurs after the seventh nerve, the nerve of the face muscles, is cut in " Bell's Palsy ".

What we have described applies to right-handed persons who are left-brained, who have aphasia along with paralysis of the right hand and arm.

A left-sided lesion in left-handed people who are right-brained, produces right-sided limb paralysis but no aphasia, because their motor speech-centre is on the right.

A right-sided lesion in a left-handed person, of course, produces both paralysis of the left hand and aphasia.

The aphasias due to disorders in the Sensory Centres are sometimes called Amnesias ; they are due to loss of comprehension of heard or seen words. The power to speak is retained, and there is no paralysis of the muscles of articulation, but as the patient does not understand what is said to him, he cannot reply ; it is as though he had been addressed in a foreign language. This is called " Wernicke's Aphasia " after the writer who devoted so much attention to it. The patient is word-deaf, and can make no appropriate reply to a question, for he has not understood it.

Occasionally word-deafness is found as a congenital defect because of the non-development of the heard word-centre; the child in consequence grows up so extremely stupid that he finds himself greatly handicapped at school.

When the centre for the comprehension of the seen word is the seat of the lesion, the patient cannot read either to himself or aloud, a condition called Alexia. You give him a newspaper upside down and he holds it so, pretending to read, for these people do not like to appear to be uneducated.

The sensory speech centres in right-handed people are found only in the left hemisphere; so that the potential centres in the right hemisphere have to be laboriously educated if the lesion on the left is of a permanent nature.

But ideas can be expressed in writing as well as by spoken words; and education consists in the training of a writing centre called, on the suggestion of Bastian, the Cheiro-kinæsthetic centre, the centre for the memories of the movements of the hand. This in right-handed persons is a left-sided centre. The writing centre informs the motor centres (Ferrier's) for the muscles of the hand, just as the motor speech-centre informs Ferrier's centres for the muscles of articulation.

It is evident that in learning originally to write, we used the visual word-centre in conjunction with the writing centre (copying), and that in writing to dictation we used the heard word-centre and the writing centre.

But a lesion of the visual word-centre will render a patient incapable of copying a MS; and a lesion of the heard word-centre will make him incapable of writing to dictation (Agraphia). All these conditions are known in neurological practice.

It is perfectly possible to lose the power of comprehension of heard or seen words and yet retain the understanding of other acquisitions such as musical notation, algebra, Hebrew, which involved the learning of special visual forms. This fact was one of those originally noted by Gall and used by him to support the view that mental acquisitions, in that they could thus be gained and lost independently of one another, must have separate cerebral localizations, which was a perfectly legitimate physiological inference.

The "deaf-and-dumb alphabet" is a conventional pantomime of great usefulness in deaf-mutism. It is, however, possible to teach the deaf-and-dumb to speak, although the process is an exceedingly laborious one. The method is as follows: two or three fingers of the dumb child's hand are placed over the larynx of the teacher, who at the same time places his mouth in the position for producing one of the vowels, for instance $\overline{\text{oo}}$, which he phonates slowly and distinctly. The child detects by the sense of touch the vibrations of the teacher's vocal cords; and at the same time, imitating the teacher, he puts his own mouth into the position for saying $\overline{\text{oo}}$. After a little while the child is able to say $\overline{\text{oo}}$. The procedure for the other sounds is similar. In this laborious manner these children can be trained to speak. Their voices have a curiously unpleasant, impersonal character because the children, being deaf, are quite unable to correct any intonational faults.

In the case of deaf-mutes taught to speak in this fashion, instead of a heard word-centre, a centre peculiar to themselves is being trained. It is a sensory centre for perceiving the vibrations of the vocal cords; we might call it the laryngo-vibrational centre.

Lastly there are children born blind and deaf whom it has actually been found possible to train to speak. The method is as described for the deaf-mutes by making them feel the vibrations of the teacher's larynx but with this addition, that simultaneously they have to feel the vibrations of their own. The fingers of one hand are placed on the teacher's thyroid cartilage, those of the other over the patient's own ; in this way these blind deaf-mutes train their laryngo-vibrational centre to instruct their latent speech centre, with the amazing result that these children can actually be taught to speak, although they never hear a word that they or other people say.

I knew one such case at the "School for the Deaf" in Halifax, Nova Scotia, where a blind boy, a deaf-mute since three months old, was taught to speak by the vibrational method. He was then ten years old ; and both his vocal acquirements and general intelligence were amazing.

The name of Helen Keller is the best known of these cases : this blind deaf-mute was taught to speak, and soon exhibited a considerable degree of intellectual power.

CHAPTER XI

PAIN; AND ITS VARIETIES

Pain may be described as a disagreeable variety of sensation which we desire to terminate. We distinguish bodily pain from mental pain, but in a sense all pain is mental in that it requires a certain degree of consciousness in order to be perceived at all; for, no brain, no pain.

We have a good deal of evidence that there are in some parts of the body nerves of "pure" pain—that is, nerves whose stimulation gives rise only to pain.

The sensations for which the skin is responsible are touch, heat, cold and pain. These may be tested for by the use of a metal rod (like a pencil) ground to a not-too-sharp point which is pressed vertically on the skin. Beginning with the rod at the temperature of the body, and exploring an area of skin in this way, we may get any of the following sensations—contact, heat, cold or "no response". When this last is reported, if we now increase the pressure very slightly, a distinct pain is suddenly developed. The nerve-endings for these various skin sensations are disposed in a punctate[1] manner, and we are stimulating mechanically the nerve-endings for pain in the skin. The cornea—very specialized skin—is a tissue which has nerves only of pure pain.

To test the absence of superficial pain in a patient, a perfectly clean needle may be made to transfix a fold of the skin ; but to investigate the painfulness of deeper structures a specially designed instrument must be used which registers the amount of the pain-producing pressures employed.

Pain, as a term, indicates a number of very different conditions. We speak of toothache being painful, we say that a particular juxtaposition of colours is " positively painful ", and we talk of the pain of parting, and of a painful duty to perform. As regards physical pain, it may be taken as certain that no pain can be felt unless a nerve is involved in the process ; thus persons afflicted with leprosy, in whom the nerves of the fingers have degenerated, can have their fingers burnt,

[1] Punctate means that the receptors for cutaneous sensations are disposed after the manner of points or dots and not in networks.

crushed, or scalded without experiencing the slightest inconvenience whatsoever.

(1) The first species of physical pain is due to normal stimuli reaching nerve-fibres in an abnormal manner; under which head fall all such pains as those from cuts, burns, lacerations, stabs, gunshot wounds, and all irritations of exposed nerves. The pain due to the familiar corn is an example of nerve-fibres being stimulated directly, for the fine, sharp, downwardly directed processes of horn (which constitute the corn) are by pressure on the surface driven into the delicate network of nerve fibrils in the true skin. So far as consciousness is concerned, it is as if the nerve had been stabbed by some foreign body like a needle or the sting of an insect. The very familiar pain of toothache is due to the mechanical stimulation of the naked fibrils of the dental nerves which have been irritated by the presence of food particles, hot or cold water, or even air having gained access to them by the decay and removal of the protecting dentine.

(2) The next species of pain is that due to excessive stimulation of sensory end-organs, as for instance the pain of an extremely bright light, a screeching, penetrating sound,

extremes of heat or cold, great pressures and so forth.

We are far from understanding what it is makes one pain " burning ", another " tearing ", and another " stabbing ". What it is that underlies a " dull " pain and makes it quite different in consciousness from a " sharp " pain, we cannot tell.

(3) Passing from pains that are virtually abnormal or pathologically intense sensations, we come to a group of pains related to organs which in health are not represented in consciousness at all. In perfectly healthy conditions of body we are not aware of any of the following—heart, pleura, stomach, intestines, liver, gall-bladder, bile-duct, spleen, kidneys, ureter, or of the periosteum, the membrane covering the bones. In other words, perfect health means that our consciousness is not occupied with the normal state or activity of our internal organs; for, as has been well said, the healthy man does not know he has a stomach or a liver. But in proportion as the states of these organs are not normal, they affect consciousness at first as uneasiness, then as discomfort, and finally as actual pain. Thus, taking the case of the heart; normally,

stimulation of its afferent nerves never enters consciousness, in other words it has afferent but not sensory nerves. But if the circulation through the heart becomes defective or locally abolished, then the state known as *angina pectoris* is set up, accompanied by what has been described as the most awful pain which any one can be called upon to suffer.

Normally we are not aware of the presence of the liver, gall-bladder, or bile-duct. But in the event of a gall-stone having entered the duct, then the muscle of that tube contracts so violently upon the resistant body that a most painful state—biliary colic—is brought on. The pain is sickening and exhausting in a high degree. This, then, is an example of "pure" or visceral pain. The colics resulting from dietetic indiscretions are pains arising from spasms of the muscular coats of the stomach and intestine which are endeavouring to reduce to pulp the too resistant masses within them. Excessive pressures on nerve-fibres for pure pain are the physical basis of this order of visceral pain.

Our last example of pure pain may be taken from the inflammation of the periosteum, the membrane covering the bones. When normal, this tissue is entirely outside our consciousness, but when inflamed in periostitis, it can give rise to pain of a persistent and torturing description.

We do not require to rely on merely indirect evidence that the healthy viscera are insensitive, for surgeons have been assured by patients who have come out of the chloroform too soon, that the manipulations of the intestines and other internal organs were painful only when the diseased regions were touched. All biologists know how the great Dr Harvey, accompanied by Charles I, visited a "Lord Montgomery", whose heart was exposed (ectopia cordis). Harvey and the King both touched the beating organ; but unless the young man watched them touch it, he was perfectly unaware that they were doing so. Still more remarkable is the fact, vouched for by men skilled in the surgery of the brain, that the removal of portions of that organ is unattended by sensation.

Closely allied to pure visceral pains we have pains associated with injuries or inflammation of the nerves themselves—neuralgias, literally nerve-pains. In a sense, as we have seen, all pains are neural; but in neuralgia the nerve-trunks themselves are the seat of the pressure or irritation. The healthy nerve-trunks no more obtrude themselves into consciousness than do the healthy viscera. Since, then, we possess normally no sensations referable to nerves in their course, and since there are pains unquestionably related to disordered conditions of nerve-trunks—neuralgia, sciatica, neuritis—it is more than probable that the "nervi nervorum" or "nerves of nerves" are for the conveyance of purely painful impulses.

On ultimate analysis these nerve-pains are due to the pressure of the blood or of lymph accumulated between the fibre-bundles and their dense inelastic sheaths, that is, congestion with pressure-effects. Why there should be a pain-perceiving mechanism in connection with our nerves is a question which physiology as such cannot answer with certainty. The subject of referred pain has been dealt with in connexion with reflex action.

The tendency to peripheral reference especially in regard to pain is well known in the case of what is called by psychologists, "the hallucination of the absent member". Suppose that a person of middle age has his leg amputated at the knee, he may suffer for years afterwards from the persistent sensation of his lost leg, and even from well-marked pain in it. Thus, as Wedgwood the famous potter found, although he underwent the amputation of a leg which had been for years a source of pain, he was not so very much benefited since he had the most distinct pain in the " absent member ". One man was known to have been tormented by a corn in the amputated foot. This phenomenon is due to the nerves involved in the " stump " sending impulses to that part of the brain in which for so many years were registered the sensations, and it may be pains, of which the absent limb *was* the origin. Thus, pain is at once truly physical and truly mental; no better example of this could be given. Of course, pain is a mental state, but it is equally a physical; the so-called " Christian scientists " have magnified the former fact to the exclusion of the latter. The great fatigue and depression which comes on after severe or prolonged suffering is unquestionably the result of damage to the sensory portions of the central nervous system.

True pain may, on several grounds, be distinguished from the many other modes of sensation, and, if this is so, it would be reasonable to suppose that pain impulses have a separate path of conduction within the spinal cord on their way to the seats of consciousness.

Neurologists believe that they have found such. It seems fairly certain that pain-producing impulses travel in a region of the spinal cord which is not shared by those of the other senses. Thus it is found that if in some kinds of accidents to the back, the lateral strands of white matter in the spinal cord have been severed, the patient retains his senses of touch and of movement, but loses the sense of pain.

This phenomenon is known as the "dissociation of the senses"; usually when the pain-sense is abolished, the senses of heat and cold are abolished along with it.

There were cases during the Great War where the injuries to the back were of such a kind that the pain-tracts were severed or pressed upon, with the result that the patient felt no pain; his skin could be cut, pinched or crushed without any discomfort. The patient could lift up red-hot coal and yet feel no pain.

There is no doubt that in an earlier and darker age, persons with this ability (or disability) were persecuted as wizards or witches in league with the Devil.

Death was the penalty of this; witches were drowned or buried alive because the physiology of the senses was not understood.[1]

That there is such a thing as pain by itself and as distinct from the sensations is corroborated by the interesting fact that in chloroform anæsthesia all the varieties of sensation are not abolished at the same time, but, on the contrary, in the following order:—the muscular sense and sense of weight, smell and taste, sight, hearing, pain and lastly the sense of contact. Thus, people "going off" have a sense of floating, or flying or sinking because their sense of weight and of movement has been abolished; they can still smell the chloroform and see and hear. Next, smell and taste vanish, but the patient can see and hear; then sight goes and then hearing. The experienced anæsthetist knows that within the next few moments pain will have been abolished although the sense of touch may still be present. Finally, this last point of contact with the outer world vanishes, and nothing more is present to consciousness.

[1] A witch was burned at Dornoch in Scotland as late as 1722.

CHAPTER XII

SLEEP, SLEEPLESSNESS AND DREAMING

Because a thing is familiar it does not follow that we know all about it. Nothing in our life is more familiar than going to sleep, and yet physiologists are by no means agreed upon what exactly determines the onset of sleep.

Sleep is the normal, recurring, resting time of the brain and mind. Complete inactivity of the brain has on its psychic side unconsciousness; and sleep is the rhythmic or phasic onset of normal unconsciousness.

Sleep has a rhythm: once every 24 hours the organ of consciousness (the cortex cerebri) rests itself; and for eight hours or so there is a complete break in the continuity of our mental and emotional life. It would seem that this resting on the part of the brain is absolutely necessary; the brain, unlike a watch, cannot go on continuously.

Dreaming is due to the partial activity of a

portion of the brain, and to that extent the refreshing unconsciousness of dreamless sleep is interfered with. About one-third of our life has to be spent in the unconsciousness of sleep, for Nature has no other method of preventing that most delicate of all her productions, the human brain, from being over-worked.

We must sleep to live ; even food cannot take the place of sleep. A sleepless animal is as miserable at the end of three to four days as a starved one at the end of ten to fifteen days. Just as the brain tissue and its correlative, consciousness, are things absolutely unique in Nature, so we find an absolutely unique method of refreshing these —" chief nourisher in Life's feast " as Shakespeare calls sleep in *Macbeth*.

Now if we analyze the conditions which predispose to sleep, we shall find four of them co-operating to that end, namely, fatigue, absence of sensations, absence of thoughts and a less energetic flow of blood through the brain.

We may allude to these four factors as the Chemical, the Sensory, the Mental and the Vascular, respectively.

On any one occasion, one of these factors

may predominate over the other three; but all co-operate in some degree to bring about the phasic state of repose of the brain.

Each of these causes of sleep is related to a type of sleeplessness or insomnia.

We shall examine these causal conditions of sleep in the order in which they have just been given.

(1) We cannot sleep unless we are tired.[1] Healthy fatigue is one of the surest conditions for inducing sleep: "The sleep of a labouring man is sweet", says the Preacher. There is no doubt that fatigue is chemically a condition of mild blood-poisoning, that as a consequence of the continuous activity of the various tissues of the body, including the nervous system itself, certain chemical substances circulate in the blood. These, it would seem, tend in some degree to poison the brain cells related to consciousness in such a fashion that they are immobilized and do not allow, as formerly, the free passage of impulses over them, the psychic correlative of which is the unconsciousness of sleep.

This chemical induction of sleep can be very striking in those cases where the fatigue

[1] This statement does not of course apply to the hypnotic trance, nor to the falling asleep of the dogs in Professor Pavlov's experiments on Inhibition.

is long continued and profound (exhaustion). As has been well said: "We stifle our brain with the ashes of our waking fires".

If fatigue is sufficiently intense, nothing can prevent the onset of sleep, as in the days of the muzzle-loaders in the "wooden walls" of old England, when a gun-crew in sheer exhaustion would lie down beside the guns, which continued the cannonade at their very ears.

Sir Philip Gibbs has described this chemical poisoning type of sleep so well in his account of the Retreat from Mons that one cannot do better than quote it—"Being attacked was the only thing that kept them awake. Towards the end of this fighting they had a drunken craving for sleep, and they slept standing, with their heads falling over the parapet; slept sitting hunched in ditches; slept like dead men where they lay on the open ground. In body and brain those men of ours were tired to the point of death. When called upon to make one last effort after six days and nights of fighting and marching, many of them staggered like men who had been chloroformed, with dazed eyes and grey, drawn faces, speechless and deaf, blind to the menace about them".

This is a marvellously accurate description of the physiological condition of men so poisoned by fatigue-products that they *must* sleep. They stagger because their motor mechanisms are poisoned, they are speechless, deaf and blind because their sensory centres are poisoned and paralyzed: nothing but sleep can revive them. They *must* sleep, army orders or no army orders.

It should be noted that it is only the higher parts of the brain, those related to consciousness, which can truly be said to sleep; the rest of the nervous system continues its activities with just a little less intensity than before.

The centre for respiration, for instance, continues to send out its rhythmic impulses to the diaphragm and to other muscles of breathing; the motor centres of the spinal cord, while not controlling the muscles so energetically, are nevertheless capable of activity. Thus it is that people can talk in their sleep, or walk in their sleep, or stand upright in their sleep as tired-out sentries have occasionally been "guilty" of doing.

The lower motor centres not being related to consciousness do not go to sleep; so that a very fatigued man can walk in his sleep along a familiar road, or swim asleep as some cross-channel swimmers have been found doing, or keep his seat on horse-back as the exhausted postillion could in the old days of the stage-coach.

This sort of thing is not quite the same as somnambulism, which is of the nature of a motor or acted dream. It is to this chemically induced type of sleep with maintenance of the posture that Shakespeare alludes when, addressing sleep, he asks—

> "Wilt thou upon the high and giddy mast
> Seal up the ship boy's eyes and rock his brains
> In cradle of the rude imperious surge ?"

Now it sometimes happens that these fatigue-products are of such a kind that instead of calming the brain-cells they irritate them, with the result that sleep is banished.

This type of insomnia is seen after *excessive* exercise, when the athlete is not "in training": children sometimes show this condition when they complain of being "too tired to sleep".

Allied to each type of sleep there is an abnormal one; and the abnormal sleep corresponding to chemically induced type is the deep sleep due to the action of the narcotic drugs of which opium and chloroform are the most familiar. The more mildly acting drugs such as the bromides we call hypnotics.

The coma of diabetes, and of kidney disease is a pathological variety of sleep closely allied to this first or chemical type.

(2) The second factor productive of sleep is a negative one, the absence of sensations. We go to sleep soonest when we retire into the dark, shut our eyes and exclude the sounds of the outer world.

Any sensory stimulation tends to keep us awake[1]; being too hot or too cold, finding the bed-clothes too light or too heavy, having cold feet or, of course, most serious of all, being in pain.

Pain and sleep are incompatible; long-continued pain is deleterious to the nervous system so that the physician does all he can to induce sleep and so prevent the pain being perceived for "he that sleeps feels not the toothache", as Shakespeare has it.

Sensations which do not vary in intensity come in time to fail to engage attention; and the brain rests so perfectly that it falls asleep. The infant falls asleep when the

[1] The exception of a monotonous sensory experience is only an apparent one, because through its monotony it ceases to be, physiologically, a stimulation.

monotonous "lullaby" is sung to it; but would be kept awake by irregular, unfamiliar noises of no greater intensity.

We fall asleep during monotonous reading or droning preaching; and we can sleep through the continuous rattle of the train; but we awake when the preacher stops or raises his voice, and when the train pulls up at a station. It is the *change* that constitutes the stimulus.

The insomnia of this sensory type of sleep is, therefore, very clearly due to the presence of sensations or of pain. The abnormal variety of sleep related to this second type is the "mesmeric" trance, a state of brain in which perception has been abolished by the induction of hypnosis—a unique condition which some would describe as inhibition of the sensory centres.

(3) The third factor inducing sleep is another negative one, the absence of emotions, thoughts, worries, etc., in a word the higher activities of the brain and mind. Thoughts we cannot banish, banish sleep; and a mind obsessed is a mind not at rest.

> "Care keeps his watch in every old man's eye;
> And where care lodges, sleep will never lie"

as we are told in *Romeo and Juliet*.

The insomnia related to the mental factor is therefore the very familiar sleeplessness owing to the persistence of thoughts—a term covering all forms of cerebral activity. The abnormal variety of sleep of this third type is the sleep of persons of very low intellectual endowment, Russian peasants for instance, who fall asleep very easily from vacancy of mind.

(4) The last causal factor of sleep is diminution of the energy of the circulation of blood in the brain. The functional activity of an organ varies with the amount of blood in it, and the brain is no exception. We have a number of proofs that just before and during sleep there is relatively less blood inside the skull than there was in the waking state.

One of the direct proofs is to allow a dog, whose skull has a trephine hole with a glass disc fitted into it, to fall sleep. Not only can one *see* that the brain is paler, but that its surface has now receded from the glass which in the waking state it was just able to touch.

Every mother knows that the membrane (the anterior fontanelle) on the top of her infant's head bulges up less during sleep than it did when the child was awake. The only position in which puppies could *not* sleep was when their heads were lower than their bodies.

Now if during sleep there is less blood in the brain, there must be more in the internal organs and the skin.

The Italian physiologist, Mosso, demonstrated this redistribution in a striking way. He placed the laboratory attendant on a horizontal hinged board like a "see-saw", and allowed him to go to sleep on it. As he fell asleep, the end of the board where the feet were began to dip, and it sank to a point indicating the displacement of 260 cc. of blood from the head end.

But without all this paraphernalia we know that there is more blood in the skin during sleep and, therefore, less in the brain because of the flushed warm skin characteristic of a sleeping person. This is the physiology of the "sleeping beauty"; children and persons with transparent skins show the flush most. A hot bath by drawing off blood into the skin is an excellent soporific.

But all the blood cut off from the brain is not accommodated in the skin; some of it goes to the digestive and other internal organs.

Thus, we know that a full meal, especially if we take it in a warm room, predisposes us to sleep. The reason is that the stomach now requires so much more blood to enable it to do its work of digestion that the brain is to that extent depleted of blood.

In the last analysis it is a question of reduced blood pressure in the cerebral arteries supplied by the carotids. The very word "carotid" comes from the rather rare Greek word *caros* ("deep sleep") from the fact well known to the ancients that by compression of the carotids unconsciousness could be produced. This method of anæsthesia was used regularly in the East even before the time of Galen to bring about a painless condition in preparation for the rough surgical operations of the time.

The abnormal state of the brain related to the vascular sleep-producing factor is the unconsciousness of fainting, of severe bleeding whether external or internal, of a very feebly acting heart and of the low blood-pressure which characterizes certain diseases.

The sleeplessness arising from the vascular factor is very evidently an excited state of the heart which, pumping too much blood through the brain, keeps it awake.

The fact that this fast action of the heart may have had an emotional origin does not make this any the less a vascular phenomenon.

The treatment of this kind of insomnia is very clear: calm the heart and lower the blood pressure in the brain. A warm bath, even only a foot-bath, taken just before bed-time, often produces the same result. A glass of warm milk many find a good soporific.

The resemblances between sleep and death, so emphasized by the poets, are quite superficial and have no physiological sanction. In this respect the poets have not displayed that intuition of scientific truth for which in so many other instances they have been conspicuous.

A dream is the arousing of some degree of consciousness during sleep. It is the psychic result of some activity in a sensory centre during sleep. A dream is mental activity during sleep, hence in the profoundest sleep we do not dream. Inasmuch as we dream, we are tending towards the reviving of consciousness; and some dreams are so vivid as actually to waken the sleeper. It is believed that the majority of dreams occur during the time when sleep is becoming less and less deep; although we have abundant evidence that dreaming can occur during the converse process of falling asleep. The famous case of this is that of the man who blew the candle out, and, having dreamt he had travelled round the world, awoke to find the wick of the candle still red.

As physiologists, we have every right to assert that the physical basis of a dream is the functional activity of a part of a sensory cerebral centre. If we take the ordinary vision or dream in which the visual centre is involved, we shall have a concrete case before us.

In healthy, sound sleep the centre for vision sees nothing because the eyes being shut, no nerve-impulses are reaching the brain from the retina. Physiologically, the dream of seeing something (visual dream) is due to the partial activity of the visual centre at a time when the rest of the centre is, as it should be, in repose.

When a centre is in activity at a time when its appropriate sense-organ is not, we call the result in consciousness a " hallucination ". In plainer language, when we see something and there is nothing corresponding to the vision to feel or handle, we are experiencing a hallucination. The classical case of a hallucination of vision in the waking state is the famous dagger of Macbeth:

A dream involving the centre for vision, is, therefore, a visual hallucination: a dream of this kind is a sensation without that sensation having an external source.

Any dream is, then, the sensory hallucination of a sane person asleep. For there are hallucinations of the insane in their waking state, and very dangerous some of these may be.

Thus, Shakespeare's phrase, "the baseless fabric of a vision", is accurate; the fabric is baseless because the dream is produced by no external visual stimulation.

In sleep, the eyes are closed and we are generally in the dark. But in spite of there being no stimulation by light, a vision is seen because only the centre is in activity. Otherwise put, the dream is central activity without activity of the retina, the appropriate end-organ. This perception is hallucinatory. It should be understood that unless nerve-impulses traverse the visual centre, nothing whatever can be seen.

Still confining our attention to this centre, it may be asked, if the eyes are closed and we are in the dark, whence came the impulses that have aroused the centre to activity? The answer is, the impulses may have arisen in the skin and muscles, in the internal organs or in another sensory centre. Nerve-impulses which arise in the skin should, of course, proceed to the centre for registering cutaneous sensations, but that centre is asleep, and the impulses failing to enter it are shunted into the visual centre where they become the physical basis of a dream. Such impulses we call "aberrant", because they have wandered away from their own proper centre and reached the visual. They reach the visual centre because the paths into it are more accessible to impulses than are the paths into any other centre. This is because of the immense functional importance of the centre for seeing, since it is so much more constantly in use than any other sensory centre. Its activity means so much in our daily lives. More technically put, there is a high degree of canalization or facilitation in the visual centre.

Currents or impulses which thus give rise to dreams may for convenience be called oneirogenetic (from the Greek *oneiros*, a dream, and *genao*, I produce).

Cases of this kind of dream are very

common. Thus when the famous Dr Gregory went to sleep with too hot a water-bottle at his feet and dreamed that he was walking on the burning lava of Mount Etna, his visual centre had been stimulated by aberrant impulses from the skin. Changes in the temperature of the skin of the sleeper are very apt to be oneirogenetic, as when the bedclothes fall off and we dream we are in the Arctic regions, or when we have too much on the bed and dream we are scorched by a tropical sun.

A dream has come to be called a "vision" by reason of the fact that undoubtedly the vast majority of dreams are of seeing something: but the centre for hearing can also dream when sounds, voices or music may be heard.

When the stimulation of a centre by its own sense-organ produces the normal effect of activity of that centre, we call the dream an "appropriate" one; but when the centre is actuated by impulses which have not arisen in the related sense-organ, we call the dream "inappropriate". The vast majority of dreams of the visual centre are, in the nature of things, *in*appropriate, for from the closed eyes in the dark no normal stimulation of the visual centre can occur. The eyes are sense-organs which we can voluntarily protect from stimulation as when we shut our eyelids. But we cannot, unfortunately, close our ears and so cut off all external sounds.

All sorts of sounds are liable to be going on during sleep—and in modern life increasingly—which, if all heard and correctly interpreted, would mean we were already awake, so impulses set up in the auditory nerve are very liable to reach the *visual* centre and produce an inappropriate dream there. In other words, sounds, like touches, may produce visions.

In actual experience what very often happens is that when the auditory centre is primarily stimulated both it and the visual centre dream, so that we have a dream appropriate to the former but inappropriate to the latter. The following is a good example of this. The external sound was that of hammering, a car being repaired in a neighbouring garage one summer morning when the windows of the house were open. A lady, not sufficiently disturbed to be awakened, dreamt that she was one of a party at dinner in a restaurant and that she was annoyed by the presence of a woman at a table nearby who wore a bangle on her wrist which, every time she moved, struck her plate. Here the stimulus was sound, but the visual centre was in full co-operation with the hearing centre. There is no doubt that a person's own snoring can be the source of his dreams.

Both the appropriate and inappropriate type of dream is well described in *Romeo and Juliet*, where Mercutio says that Queen Mab, the fairies' midwife—

> " gallops night by night
> . . . .
> O'er lawyers' fingers who straight dream on fees,
> O'er ladies' lips who straight on kisses dream,
> . . . .
> Sometimes she gallops o'er a courtier's nose
> And then dreams he of smelling out a suit,
> And sometimes comes she with a tithe-pig's tail
> Tickling a parson's nose as a'lies asleep,
> Then dreams he of another benefice :
> Sometimes she driveth o'er a soldier's neck,
> And then he dreams of cutting foreign throats,
> Of breaches, ambuscades and Spanish blades,
> Of healths, five fathoms deep, and then anon
> Drums in his ear, at which he starts and wakes,
> And, being thus frighted, swears a prayer or two,
> And sleeps again."

The relationship between a particular stimulus and the subsequent dream was made the subject of experimentation many years ago by the Frenchman, Alfred Maury. When a pair of tweezers was made to vibrate near his ears, Maury dreamed of bells, of the tocsin and of the events of June, 1848. When his lips were tickled, he dreamt that a pitch-plaster was being torn off his face by the old doctor of his childhood. Perfumes brought close to the nostrils induced dreams of pleasant smells, as when he dreamt he was in a conservatory, and on one occasion in a well-known scent shop in Cairo. When a drop of water was placed on his forehead, Maury dreamt he was in Italy in hot weather perspiring and drinking wine. Those dreams were more "appropriate" than one might have expected.

Occasionally a wholly appropriate visual dream *is* experienced, as when a man, not wholly awakened by the rays of the rising sun, dreamed of seeing flames issuing from the mouths of dragons. One case is recorded where strong moonlight falling on the sleeper produced a dream of his embracing his lady-love—"the lady of his dreams", in fact. It has been suggested that rays of light falling into the eyes of persons in the coma of impending death may have caused them to dream of bright beings—"angels"—and so waken them and make them speak of "heaven opened".

Hitherto we have considered as oneirogenetic only impulses arising in the organs of special sense, the skin and the muscles, what for convenience we call the ecto-periphery, but it is pretty well known that currents from the internal organs (ento-periphery) may be quite as effectively dream-producing. Doubtless neither while awake nor asleep ought we to have any consciousness of the state of our internal organs beyond, of course, some hunger and a sense of well-being after a meal (coenæsthesia). But the most of us unfortunately know that in actual life this is far from being the case, for from time to time we are made painfully aware of our digestive and other internal organs. Now it is certain that impulses from the internal organs can become dream-producing. It is accepted on all hands as indisputable that a late supper will be sure to make us dream, and the " lobster salad " is regarded as singularly effective in this respect. The inactive stomach does not obtrude itself into consciousness nor does the slightly active organ dealing with a normally digestible meal, but the increased muscular activity (peristalsis) associated with an indigestible meal taken shortly before going to bed may certainly produce dreaming of a highly unpleasant character. The old notion that digestion was suspended in sleep has been proved incorrect by Pavlov's observations on sleeping dogs. Clearly the dream following on indigestion is " inappropriate ", for impulses from internal organs are gaining access to the visual centres to which they are totally alien.

And so it is with the other internal organs, the intestines, heart, liver, gall-bladder and urinary bladder, to name only a few. If the activities of any of these become at all pronounced, the impulses so aroused are extremely liable to be dream-producing.

When the disordered state of the heart is the causal condition, very distressing dreams may accompany the cardiac pain. The physician is, of course, fully aware of these facts. He does well to warn his patients that after taking a pill they may have disagreeable dreams, for the increased muscular activity occasioned by the pill is often oneirogenetic. Colic is powerfully so. A full bladder particularly in children is almost certainly the source of dreams. The lungs, too, are sometimes oneirogenetic, especially when their bronchial muscle goes into the state of spasm (asthma).

All these dreams induced by abnormal states of internal organs are apt to become coloured with unpleasant emotion and so lead to incubus or nightmare, a state in which oppression, suffocation or the inability to move, walk or run is the hallucination. In pre-scientific days, the belief was that a female evil spirit actually sat upon the chest of the sleeper and overpowered or paralyzed him. In Babylonian mythology Labartu, a horrible monster, caused nightmare and certain ills peculiar to women. In nightmare and in all dreams which are highly coloured emotionally, there is the tendency to irradiate. If the dream is in the visual centre, then the spread of nerve-impulses is into muscles, including the heart, and into various glands in a manner about which we may inquire more fully a little later on.

Allied to nightmare are the night-terrors of children. *Pavor nocturnus*, as it is called in medicine, is a vivid and highly disagreeable dream produced usually by some abnormal state of an internal organ, often colic. What used to be called " growing-pains " in children are certainly responsible for some of their nightmares. Growing-pains are now known to be an expression of rheumatism in the bones, for the growth of healthy bone is quite painless. It is probably true that if a child is at all often worried by "night-terrors", his nervous system may need critical attention, for some instability of it may be detectable.

We have seen that the visual centre is the one which most frequently dreams because of the greater degree of canalization of it than is found in any other centre. But in the case of the congenitally blind, there can be no functionally educated visual centre, so that these persons must dream in terms of sensations other than visual. One blind boy dreamed of Alexander the Great by hearing guns firing, that is, he had a purely auditory dream. (The anachronism of guns in the time of Alexander must be pardoned.) A blind man dreamed that a relative was dead by his being conscious of touching a cold corpse. Another dreamed of the "Day of Judgment" by being pulled up to Heaven by a rope and hearing trumpets sounding.

Most dreams fade away with the rapidity with which they were born. Now and again, however, the dream-images are of such a character that emotions or ideas are aroused which in their turn are expressed through the appropriate physiological mechanisms. This sort of thing we refer to as the *dream overflow*. When the dream has become invested with strong emotional colouring, the dreamer may be awakened with all the symptoms of emotional disturbance—rapid heart action (palpitation), trembling, perspiration, weeping, one or all of these. Such dreams are commoner in children than in adults, but are by no means rare at any time of life. The overflow of the nerve-energy may be into the heart, accelerating it, into the sweat glands and the tear glands, making them active, and into the body muscles, throwing them into a greater or less degree of tremor. This is the physiology of " to dream of the devil and wake in a fright " (*Ingoldsby Legends*), and of Macbeth's complaint of " these terrible dreams that shake us nightly ". A sensitive child may wake up screaming with muscles all trembling and skin bathed in perspiration. The oneirogenetic impulses in the visual centre have overflowed into such cerebral regions as are the physical bases of emotion and of " meaning ", wherever these may be, and have so roused them that through the violence of the expression of the emotions the sleep has actually been terminated.

When the overflow from the dreaming centres is into the frontal regions, the seat of the intellectual operations, then more or less definite ideas arise in the dream-consciousness. Occasionally the dreamer is amused by something seen or said in the dream and actually laughs, occasionally so loudly as to waken himself. Here the respiratory apparatus, particularly the diaphragm, is thrown into convulsive action. It is rare but not unknown to observe a sleeper smile in his sleep; healthy children may from time to time be observed to smile or laugh in their sleep.

Lastly, the dream overflow may be into the speech centres in the frontal lobes. The content of the dream may be such that it tends to induce words to be spoken so that the cerebral speech centres are energized. The term somniloquence is sometimes used for talking in sleep. The words are usually incoherent and convey no meaning to an observer, but occasionally they may be full of significance, for people have been known to make important statements in the unconsciousness of sleep. Indeed, the old Latin adage, "in vino veritas", may be paraphrased into "in somno veritas". In the dreaming that is accompanied by talking in sleep there is the same absence of reticence and abolition of conventional restraint as there is in alcoholic intoxication, so that the truth is sometimes inadvertently revealed in this manner. The novelists have not failed to make use of this knowledge, as when a murderer by talking in his sleep reveals important information about the crime he has committed, but in which his part is not suspected. We are here reminded of the Doctor's declaration in *Macbeth*—

> "Infected minds
> To their deaf pillows will discharge their secrets."

There is not the slightest doubt we are entitled to assume that certain animals, for instance the dog, can dream.

We are approaching the condition of the acted dream in which, in consequence of the related emotions or ideas, there is a tendency to appropriate motorial expression. The talking and laughing in dreams are of this exteriorizing quality. Occasionally a dreamer gets out of bed and proceeds to carry through a more or less complete and apparently rational series of actions. Such a person is called a somnambulist or sleep-walker. The tendency to sleep-walking is exhibited at an early age, and if it occurs at all frequently may be taken as evidence of some congenital instability of the nervous system.

This walking in sleep may, of course, lead the dreamer into some dangerous places, so that every now and again we read of persons falling downstairs or out of the window and so meeting their death. The movements of walking and the balancing of the body are carried out in complete unconsciousness, so that if a somnambulist happens to be walking in a dangerous place he can do it in safety, unaware of his peril. To awaken such a walker suddenly is the real danger. Sleep-walkers have been known to walk in safety over the roofs of houses and along the copings of high walls, and not to fall over.

Since somnambulists are unconscious, nothing they may do in the state of somnambulism is regarded by the law as of criminal nature. Such a person might make a murderous attack on some other person, but the law would not hold him guilty as there was no intent to kill nor any subsequent recollection of the killing. For on awaking, the somnambulist does not remember what has happened while he was asleep. In this respect the state of the consciousness resembles that in the hypnotic trance. The ordinary or awaking consciousness has vanished, and a subconscious state been substituted for it. Writers of fiction have utilized these facts, seeing that they are capable of highly sensational treatment.

Very occasionally persons asleep have risen from their beds and sat down to write something or to compose music as though in possession of full consciousness. Mathematicians have solved problems which had baffled them during their waking hours; poets have committed to paper verses that had "come" to them during sleep; and there is at least one case recorded of music having been so composed. The musician, Tartini, is said to have composed his "Devil's music" ("Trillo del Diavolo") in this manner. This highly unusual form of brain activity (cerebration) is of the order of somnambulism in that it is the exteriorizing of ideas coherent and intellectual rather than the mere expression of a motorial compulsion.

Coleridge asserted that the poem *Kubla Khan* was composed in his sleep.

The term " somnambulism " certainly does not describe those intellectual operations. Not sensations but ideas are being recorded, and this intellectual process involves the muscles of writing, it might be called somnographia, or, better, hypnographia.

Before leaving the subject of somnambulism, we might note that to walk or swim when sound asleep is not somnambulism. To walk asleep is not the same thing as walking in one's sleep. In walking when sound asleep no dream is being enacted; the walking is automatic through centres of the spinal cord acting independently of the sleeping brain. In walking in one's sleep, the subconsciousness of the dreaming brain is instigating the muscles of locomotion to motorial expression.

We are now in a position to try to discover the characteristics of the dream state.

In the first place, it would appear that our notions of time and space are, for the time being, abolished. We do not seem to be in our normal relationships to external realities. We do not seem to have our usual standards of reference with regard to the past, present or future or to the ordinary limitations of space. The most noticeable obliteration in dreaming is that of the appreciation of the flight of time. Actions which would take hours, days or years to develop seem to occur with absurd rapidity, in fact in "no time". Our familiar external standard of time is gone. The external world has been completely shut out and, as it were, forgotten, so that we do not seem to be related to any objective standards.

We behold a long-dead relative and even converse with him without the least astonishment that he has returned to life; unmoved we see him exactly as we may last have known him a generation ago. In the dream we take everything at its face value, everything for granted; we criticize nothing, are surprised at nothing, ashamed of nothing. There is nothing too absurd to be accepted at its own value, nothing too bizarre to astonish us. We are spectators of rather than participators in the weird scenes presented to our inward eye. The extreme *bizarrerie* is doubtless due to the extraordinary way in which the nerve-impulses must be wandering about undirected and uncontrolled in the sensory centres.

It is the power of criticism rather than the faculty of logical analysis that has been paralyzed. The precise physiological reason for this may be the fact that those regions of the brain believed to be the material substratum of memory, judgment and the intellectual processes in general, are inactive, so that the hallucinatory perceptions which constitute the dream are not subjected to that critical examination to which they would be in the waking state. The hallucinations are accepted as having all the validity of the reality of external things. The familiar standards of time and space given us by happenings external to us are, for the time being, gone. We have no conscious relations to past, present or future, and are disoriented or not oriented at all to the limitations of tri-dimensional space. Our introspection is complete.

The dream is thus closely allied to the insane state in which the lunatic mistakes his hallucinations for happenings which possess a basis in external reality. The dream is emphatically not a succession of memory images, although some dreams are built up around a nucleus of such images. It has been remarked that the more intellectual the person, the less of mere memories will there be in his dream. Marie de Mauaĉeïne remarks how very seldom a dreamer is confronted with his own image.

The ability to recall dreams varies from the greatest difficulty to the greatest ease. Sometimes on awaking we can scarcely recollect anything of our dream even when greatly desiring to do so, and at other times we cannot forget it even if ever so anxious. We may be " haunted by that dream " for days or weeks. The difficulty of recalling the usual sort of dream is no doubt due to the fact that the physical trace (engram) is so slight that the corresponding psychosis is very feeble, whereas the dream we cannot forget has been one that aroused emotion, meaning or interest to such an extent that it acquired some element of stability. Certain dreams may be so vivid, so reasonable, and so " sensible " that a person subsequently may be heard to remark: " Did I see that or only dream it? "—eloquent testimony to the verisimilitude of the dream.

The tendency to-day is to regard the dream-consciousness as an emergence from the subconscious mind. Someone has said the discovery of the subconscious mind by the late mystic and poet, F. W. H. Myers, was one of the great achievements of Victorian psychology.

This view accentuates the great differences between the waking consciousness and the dream consciousness. They are clearly different things, the one is by no means an extension of the other. To regard these as separate streams is to explain how, as a rule, what occurs in the one state is not remembered in the other. This has a parallel in the two aspects of personality, the ego and the alter ego; the one does not remember the deeds of the other.

Freud, as is well known, lays a great deal of stress on the contents of dreams and on their rising into consciousness when the inhibiting power of the latter has been withdrawn. Freud believes that many disagreeable and unpleasant memories are buried in our subconsciousness whence they emerge during dreaming into the conscious realm. The dream may be regarded as a kind of half-way house between the subconscious and the conscious realms. The dream consciousness not being subjected to the criticism associated with the perception of external reality, is more or less a law unto itself.

From the analysis of the dream-content, Freud has derived a very great deal of the fabric of his psycho-analytic building.

According to him, the suppressed, disagreeable or unsatisfied vicious desires or tendencies emerge from the realm of the subconscious usually under some kind of symbolic disguise.

While, of course, cases of this kind occur, it is equally true that very often in dreaming the disagreeable actualities of waking life are left behind, and for a brief space we survey, if not enjoy, " scenes that are brighter ". The world forgetting, we live for a little, if not exactly in " the freshness ", then in " the glory of a dream ".

There seems no reason to doubt that persons while dreaming have received information of a more or less definite kind, which was of vital import for them. This information is conveyed telepathically, that is directly to the brain without having been communicated through the sleeper's organs of sense. From the earliest times, messages, warnings, exhortations and revelations have come in dreams. When the future was divined through dreams in a systematic manner, the term " oneiromancy " was used.

Some of these dream experiences reported in our own day have been quite remarkable.

One aspect of the dream we have not yet touched on is the so-called "atavistic". By this is meant that the dream is the expression of an ancestrally derived memory. The notion is that dreams of flying or falling, for instance, are subconscious survivals of the day when our ancestors were arboreal creatures, and swung from branch to branch and leapt from the branches to the ground.

On similar lines—as unconscious or latent memory—is explained the sort of dream that we find shared, say, by father and son, or by mother and daughter.

Cases of the familial dream are by no means unknown. That some dreams are the expression of ancestral memories is an attractive theory. It assumes the inheritance of non-material, psychic traits in a subconscious manner, which is not by any means an extravagant hypothesis.

CHAPTER XIII

THE PHYSICAL BASES OF CONSCIOUSNESS

All investigators competent to pronounce upon this difficult subject have come to the conclusion that consciousness has as its physical basis the cells and synapses of the cortex cerebri and perhaps also of the optic thalamus.

By "consciousness" we understand the mental awareness of the existence of oneself and of one's environment. Consciousness as a function of brain is multiform, and has the following modes or modifications—sensations, perceptions, emotions, volitions, memories.

The three main primary divisions of mental activity are—sensations, emotions and volitions.

The evidence that the cortex cerebri is the anatomical "locus" of consciousness is full and varied. The brain, as Bastian put it, is " the organ of the mind ".

I. First of all we have the broad morphological consideration that according as there is more grey matter, the person is the more intellectual. Conversely, deficiency of intellect goes with a small amount of cortex. The term " microcephalic idiot " is applied to a well-known type of person who because he has so little grey matter has much less than the normal mentality.

Let it be noted that we say nothing about the size of the head as a whole : a small head may contain a brain with *relatively* much cortex. It is the depth and cellular richness of the cortex that is important. The cortex in man is not smooth, but is thrown into folds (convolutions) with, therefore, depressions (sulci) between them : and it is the extent of these convolutions that is so remarkable at the post mortem examination of persons of outstanding mental capacity like Gauss the mathematician, Sir James Simpson, and Helmholtz.

On surveying the animal kingdom we can say that the more intelligent the animal the better marked are its convolutions ; the less intelligent, the less well marked.

Thus, the monkey, elephant and dog belong to the former, the guinea-pig and frog to the latter group.

Further, when the cortex cerebri is absent altogether (as in congenital acephaly), the "monster", as it is called, is without any mind whatever, and for the short time it survives merely performs some bulbar reflex actions, sucking being one of them.

The first condition or basis of consciousness is, then, a morphological and quantitative one—the presence and number of cortical neurons.

II. It will, however, be apparent that consciousness does not "reside" in the neurons—this expression is at present used only for brevity—until they have attained to a certain degree of histological differentiation. They must have attained to a certain degree of cellular complexity before consciousness can become related to them. While they are as yet embryonic there is no consciousness, no memory of events, hence, we do not remember being in the womb, nor, as a matter of fact, hardly anything for the next two years. The organ is too simple for the task of registration.

Fig. 14 shows the progressive differentiation

of form and increase in complexity in the cerebral neurons as life advances. Only when they have attained to a certain internal complexity can there be, apparently, what we call memory, or revivability of impressions.

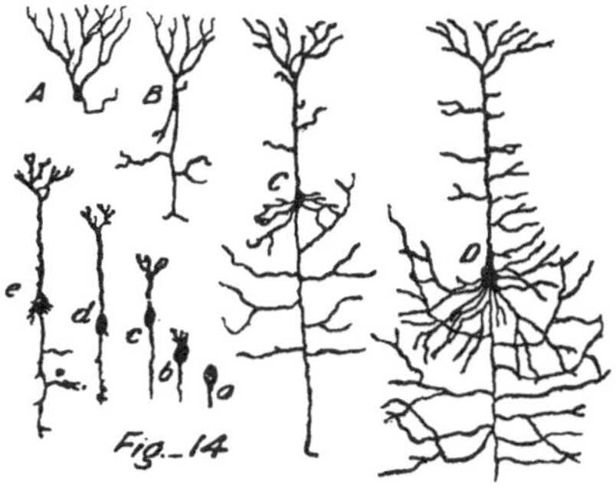

Four types of Neuron from the grey matter of the brain of frog, reptile lower mammal, man, showing ascending degrees of complexity (A-D).
Stages in the development of a single neuron from the grey matter of the brain (*a-e*).
(From Stewart's *Manual of Physiology*).

This second factor is, then, degree of differentiation. The cerebral neurons in man continue to "grow", to become more complex, up to middle life or about the fortieth year. As old age comes on we find the brain-cells showing signs of "wear and tear", of physiological atrophy, and the mind becoming concomitantly affected. Under the microscope the cells manifest some or all of the following changes: the nucleus shrivels, pigment becomes deposited in the cells, the processes atrophy. This is the physical basis of senility.

III. The third factor underlying the presence of consciousness is histological integrity. This can be compromised in several ways, and first of all by concussion. It is well known that a fall on the head or a blow on the head can make consciousness vanish. The neurons of the cortex terminate in extremely delicate, elongated, semi-fluid, protoplasmic threads interlacing with others of like tenuity forming the "synapses" of inconceivably fine structure, so that it is not in the least surprising that the violent mechanical jar we call "concussion" should dislocate these delicate mechanisms.

The living arborescence at the termination of a neuron may be likened to the tentacles of a sea-anemone expanded in the water of the tank in the aquarium. If you give a sharp tap to the glass plate of the tank, the tentacles are immediately withdrawn and curled up. There is no doubt that the limits of physical insult which these delicate synapses can withstand are easily over-passed. The high explosives used in modern warfare develop concussing power far beyond what the cell-processes of the human brain can endure. The effects of the violent mechanical injury are generally referred to as " shell-shock ".

The unconsciousness which ushers in the train of symptoms of this condition is the immediate result of the vibrational injury to the cells of the grey matter. The more permanent results may be far-reaching.

An analogous condition in the spinal cord —engine-driver's disease—is set up by the continual vibration conveyed from the foot-plate into the man's central nervous system.

Compression is another mechanical agency which can affect the central nervous system, the neurons cannot perform their functions if pressed upon unduly.

The sources of compression are of various kinds such as a depressed bone, a foreign body under the skull, a brain tumour, or an abscess. In the earlier stages, compression may act as a mechanical stimulus to the brain-cells and give rise to convulsions by the pressure on motor centres, but prolonged intra-cranial pressure is always in the end a depressant.

IV. The physico-chemical integrity of the

nerve-cell depends upon a certain upper limit of temperature not being exceeded.

In the mammal this temperature is 47° C (116° F), which is exactly the temperature at which one of the chemical constituents in the nerve-cell coagulates. At this temperature the cell is killed. This temperature, 116° F, is about 8 degrees above the highest fever temperature known (108° F). If the temperature of the blood rises to anywhere near this height, irreparable damage is done to some of the cells, and consciousness is to that extent compromised. A nerve-cell so killed is never replaced. The heat of high fever always tends to injure the cortical neurons, and we know that consciousness is pathologically altered in the delirium of high fever.

When the temperature of the blood rises to a dangerous height from the action of extreme heat, whether of the sun or otherwise, unconsciousness sets in and the condition is called "heat-stroke". A "sunstroke" is the name given to that condition of heat-damaged brain which results in a permanent alteration of mentality. Very often the mind is left slightly enfeebled in certain of its activities. A person who has had a " touch of the sun " may be peculiar or " queer " for the rest of life.

Heat, then, is an agency which by injuring the chemical condition of the brain-cells is responsible for the concomitant alteration of consciousness.

V. The next condition on which consciousness depends is the blood-supply to the brain.

We have already seen how very abundant is the blood supply to the cortex cerebri.

The whole meaning of the anastomosis of the arteries at the base of the brain (circle of Willis) is to ensure that the blood-supply of no region of the brain shall be cut off by the blocking of any one of its constituent vessels. Deprivation of blood is the most rapid way of producing unconsciousness. The blood pressure has only to fall below a certain amount for a second or two to ensure fainting with its concomitant of " the mind becoming a blank ". In fainting, the heart, for some reason or another, has failed to empty itself into the arteries for the space of a beat or two, with the result that the blood-pressure falls in those few seconds to a point incompatible with consciousness. The muscles become toneless, because imperfectly innervated, and the person falls down,

The low blood pressure entails depriving the nerve-cells of oxygen, for it is really in the last analysis lack of oxygen which is so bad for them. One object of the circulation is to supply the cells of the body with oxygen.

Similarly, a low blood-pressure brought about by a great diminution of the volume of blood in consequence of serious bleeding —external or internal—causes loss of consciousness through oxygen want. Thus the severely wounded soldier becomes unconscious on the battle-field, and may be picked up for dead.

Short of fainting, consciousness may be temporarily lost when for any reason the cerebral blood pressure is reduced.

It is here that the stimulant properties of alcohol are found useful. A tight abdominal bandage is helpful in circumstances where the blood-pressure tends to fall, as when people have to stand a long time in the heat without food. It is well known how busy the ambulance is kept at these times removing people who have fainted.

One way to revive a fainting person is to press the head between the knees: the compression thus exerted on the abdominal veins forces the stagnant blood towards the heart and so restores the pressure in the brain.

VI. The last factor underlying consciousness is the chemical state of the blood. Consciousness can be made to vanish by the inhaling of nitrous oxide, chloroform, ether and many other chemical substances.

The exact cause of unconsciousness is in all probability once most the reaction of the delicate processes at the synapses, because these are by far the most vulnerable places of the neuronic chains. Just as the tentacles of the sea-anemone will be withdrawn when some noxious material is stirred in to the water of the tank, so probably the extremely fragile living arborescences of the nerve-cells are similarly affected. We have some evidence that the cerebral neurons have retained the power of a certain degree of movement. There is histological evidence, from the brains of animals killed in this kind of chemically induced unconsciousness, that there has been some retraction of the dendrites.

In the analogous condition of very deep sleep there is also some evidence of a similar state of things.

This chemical poisoning of cerebral neurons

is of course the cause of unconsciousness in acute alcoholic intoxication. The sleep of extreme fatigue and the comas of diabetes and of other abnormal states, are, as we have seen, some examples of unconsciousness due to the operation of a chemical factor.

We have learned, then, that the maintenance of consciousness normally requires a particular normal chemical constitution of the blood, and that certain alterations of this are accompanied by corresponding alterations in the quality of the conscious states related thereto.

As to the precise "seat" of consciousness, Professor W. MacDougall, F.R.S., has made an effort to arrive at a conclusion. He believes that it is concerned with the synapses rather than the cell-bodies. This is not the place to follow him into the full discussion of the subject, but here it may be sufficient to say that his main reason for deciding on the synapses is that they are the places where changes in the resistance to the flow of impulses may pre-eminently occur.

It is empirically true that consciousness can be maintained only in so far as there are changes in the volume and intensity of the impulses flowing over the synapses, if we may be allowed to put it in such terms. When the flow is zero or minimal, unconsciousness (sleep) supervenes. When the flow is unaltered in intensity for long periods (monotonous reading, droning preaching, etc.), it ceases to be a stimulus to the cerebrum which goes to sleep. This is comparable with the well-known non-stimulating power of a galvanic current of constant intensity traversing a muscle.

The question is often asked, can consciousness exist apart from a brain or a body. Put in that form to the physiologist, he can only answer: "Not in my experience". His attitude is absolutely agnostic, all he can say is he never knew of consciousness disembodied; and he knows of no evidence for such a belief. He dare not deny that it might be, but so far as the evidence of his senses goes, he has no knowledge of it. It is difficult to conceive how a disembodied consciousness could inform an inquirer as to its existence, or even begin to communicate with him.

The relationships of mind and matter are the supreme mystery of life.

INDEX